Myron J. Stolaroff

# THANATOS TO EROS

Reihe *Ethnomedizin und Bewußtseinsforschung*
herausgegeben von Dr. Christian Rätsch

Series *Ethnomedicine and the Study of Consciousness*
edited by Dr. Christian Rätsch

## The Author

Myron J. Stolaroff was born in Roswell, New Mexico, August 20, 1920. He graduated from Stanford University in 1941 with great distinction. A year later he got his Masters Degree in electrical Engineering. After World War II he worked for Ampex Corporation as a design engineer and eventually became the Director of Instrumentation Marketing. From 1960 to 1970 he was the President of the International Foundation for Advanced Study. During that period he was the executive administrator for a research group conducting clinical studies with LSD and mescaline. He co-authored many of the Foundation staff papers on psychedelic therapy. After 1970 he worked as a Consulting Engineer and as a General Manager of Multi-Media Productions, a manufacturer of social studies and sound filmstrips for public school. He retired in 1979 to focus on personal studies. He published professional papers in the *Journal of Nervous and Mental Disease, Gnosis* and the *Yearbook for Ethnomedicine and the Study of Consciousness.* At present he serves as a member of the Board of Directors of the Albert Hofmann Foundation.

Myron J. Stolaroff

# THANATOS TO EROS

## THIRTY-FIVE YEARS OF PSYCHEDELIC EXPLORATION

VWB - Verlag für Wissenschaft und Bildung

**Coverdesign by** Jean Stolaroff

Die Deutsche Bibliothek – CIP-Einheitsaufnahme

**Stolaroff, Myron J.:**
Thanatos to Eros : thirty-five years of psychedelic exploration /
Myron J. Stolaroff. - Berlin : VWB, Verl. für Wiss. und
Bildung, 1994
(Reihe Ethnomedizin und Bewusstseinsforschung)
ISBN 3-86135-453-5

**Publisher:**
VWB – Verlag für Wissenschaft und Bildung
Amand Aglaster • P.O.Box 11 03 68 • D-10833 Berlin
Markgrafenstr. 67 • D-10969 Berlin
Phone 030 / 251 04 15 • Fax 030 / 251 04 12

**Printed in Germany by:**
GAM-Media GmbH, Berlin

# Table of Contents

# Forword

by Alexander T. Shulgin and Ann Shulgin

The search for a relationship with the universal reality about us is one of the most important goals in human life. It has to be conducted by two entirely distinct processes which, while concurrent, are totally different. The passage through your lifetime of eighty to a hundred years (give or take a few decades) involves learning relationships – giving and taking – with those who share your journey on this planet. And, at the same time, you play a role at this moment of human history. Living your own personal life in the immediate present, you are also, to an often unknowable extent, a contributor to the structure of the world about you.

Myron Stolaroff has given us an autobiography, a tale of psychological and spiritual evolution that subtly brings together these two threads, these two roles; he is both the struggling seeker for wholeness in himself, and a discoverer of new paths to wholeness for others.

The story of *Thanatos to Eros* takes us through two marriages, over the course of the author's growth from a successful engineer to an independent business man, and eventually, we see his first steps and subsequent strides as a researcher and explorer of human consciousness. We move with him through the often intense and difficult changes that take place as he learns to use his chosen tools, the psychedelic drugs, beginning with LSD in 1956, and progressing to other powerful visionary plants and drugs over the subsequent years. He is trying to, in the words of Carl Jung, "make the unconscious conscious", as the way to attain realization of his ultimate self. We discover, along with him, that this is a hard goal to attain, and that it must be sought with complete inner integrity and fearless self-examination.

Spun into the narrative are reports of some extraordinary experiences, brought about by the use of appropriate psychedelic drugs. As Stolaroff learns himself, he gains in understanding of others who are suffering pain and self-rejection, and begins to guide friends who come to him in trouble, through carefully controlled and monitored psychedelic sessions. Needless to say, since the imposition of draconian laws in recent years, this kind of deep spiritual work, done with the aid of psychedelic materials, is no longer possible, and will remain forbidden until the public is better informed and directs its lawmakers to change such restrictions on these kinds of drugs.

*Thanatos to Eros*, in the meantime, will serve the general reader and would-be researcher by defining the guidelines for the proper and safe use of psychedelic drugs in therapy and in spiritual growth. It gives us not only many beautifully presented glimpses of psychedelic experiences as they are undergone by family members and friends, but also allows us to follow the further development of many of these people in the months and years following their life-changing sessions.

Psychedelic experiences are not uniformly positive, as serious researchers know only too well. The psyche has its own agenda, and it includes exposure to places in the soul where sorrow and hopelessness reign supreme, where death stares implacably into the inner eyes, and only immense courage will bring the person through the dark tunnel and return him to light and livingness. Myron Stolaroff describes several of these difficult sessions, helping us understand that they can be of immense value in someone's spiritual progress, especially if they are shared with a guide who "knows the territory", and can help in the emotional working through of the fear and sadness that have come to the surface.

But the true treasure of this writing is the subtle message it offers the reader, as to the process of becoming a man of wisdom. All cultures through human history have respected the teacher, the shaman, the priest, and the curandero who has been available to his community, his extended family. Every society has its elders, its mavens, the wise, experienced and intuitive men and women who can offer answers to problems, counsel to the troubled, and medicine to the sick. They have lived long enough to have achieved certain levels of comprehension, to have seen connections between cause and effect, to have perceived the changes wrought by time. They have a form of knowing called wisdom.

However, it's a simple fact that the wise man, in his heart, doesn't know that he is a wise man; he is aware only of what he does not understand, cannot do, and does not yet know. He will often acknowledge having come to be more and more at peace with his immediate world, and perhaps having caught a glimpse of another world, an extended reality. His answers to anxious questions have become increasingly direct and to the point. He no longer wastes time – his own or others' – as he used to in the past, and his life is increasingly involved with a continuing process of integrating information, both consciously and subconsciously.

In Myron Stolaroff, we have a gentle, giving person who has become a helper, and guide and rescuer to many about him, but who does not see himself as an elder of the tribe, a shaman, a wise man. This is the metaphor which is the second message of this remarkable book. Enjoy the day to day narratives, and the drug experiences (mostly joyful, some difficult) that contribute to the developing relationship between participants. But also follow the gradual evolution of an imaginative and intelligent person into a wise man who begins coming to peace with himself. It is a beautiful story.

This process of personal growth and understanding could just as well have involved Buddhist practices of meditation, or training in shamanic plant medicines, or any one of innumerable other methods of achieving wholeness. It so happens that, for this good man, psychedelic drugs have been the vehicle, and it is clear that they have served him well.

It was said by Lao Tse some 25 centuries ago: "Understanding others is wisdom. Understanding yourself is enlightenment". This book is a unique illustration of what was meant by that great sage, and will enrich the inner world of the reader.

# Preface

Sigmund Freud has postulated that there lies within each of us a drive for death. As we see the self-destructive tendency operating wide-spread throughout humankind, it is easy to accept the reality of such a drive. I have certainly found it functioning with great strength within myself.

This book is the story of how I overcame thanatos, the drive for death, to elicit eros, the drive for life.

The informed use of psychedelic substances has been a key element in my personal growth. The material presented here is not intended in any way to encourage the use of illicit substances. Nor for that matter, the uninformed use of any substance, licit or illicit. The substances described in this book are powerful, and can easily be misused. They should be employed only with integrity and a thorough knowledge of their characteristics, both benefits and adverse affects.

I believe these pages contain ample evidence to support the value and usefulness of such substances. I hope that this evidence will encourage rational efforts toward further scientific exploration of these materials and the establishment of procedures to take advantage of their remarkable potential.

I am confident that in time, we will learn to use psychedelic substances to explore many aspects of science, art, history, psychology, and spirituality. The dimensions of the mind that can be realized are limited only by our willingness to enter them; eons of fascinating exploration await us.

Curious investigators focus on the particular areas that appeal to them. I have confined my own explorations within the framework of two major paradigms: psychotherapy and spirituality. My motivation is simple. Most of my life I have experienced very uncomfortable feelings. My primary motivation is simply to feel good. To accomplish this, I found great assistance through understanding my own personal psychic dynamics. This taught me to comprehend my values and behavior, and what I could do to achieve a more comfortable, satisfying, fulfilling life.

Even more helpful was my willingness to discover and draw upon the essential healing forces of the universe. By focusing on the innate life force, I found it possible to realize a level of wisdom, understanding, and universal love that I had not previously known possible.

Consequently my personal explorations generally focused on spiritual development.

Many other avenues of exploration are possible, and some of them show up in the experiences reported here. As psychedelic substances are better understood, the eager, dauntless explorers of modern times will range over these new, uncharted seas, and return with great treasures.

Names and locations have been fictionalized in this report to protect personal privacy.

Some of the characters described are composites of individuals.

## Acknowledgments

I am deeply indebted to many dear friends for making the personal adventure described in this book possible. There are wise ones who provided counsel and guidance, companions who shared deeply in the processes reported here, and courageous individuals willing to explore with little-known substances to extend our knowledge.

Extremely important for me personally have been those intimate friends in special groups who provided a centering, stabilizing force for accurate perception. A major danger in psychedelic use is to become enamored with one's own inner, subjective experience. Often exploring alone in a remote area, I sometimes gave undue weight to such creations. I was frequently rescued from erroneous conclusions by recognizing the accuracy and ingenuity of the perceptions of my companions. I'm especially grateful for this most important discovery:

I find the most enjoyable, stimulating, and fulfilling state in which to function is within the common meeting place of minds.

# Introduction

There is a light that glows continuously in the universe. It is eternal, ever-present, and unending. This light is the source of life. It can be for each of us the source of joy, wellbeing, aliveness, in fact that which makes everything in life charged with exuberance and gratitude at the miracle of being. We can be filled with wonder and excitement at participating in the enormous adventure of life. This light is infinitely expressive, constantly seeking ways to manifest in ever-unfolding, ever-increasing varieties of expression. Participating in this process brings us untold joy and delight.

We, humankind, have the opportunity to be the channel for the expression of this light. As the most developed creatures on the planet, we have been granted attributes which permit us to unite our inner self with this indescribably beautiful light, to be an expression of this energy, and to share in the joy and delight of the unfolding processes of Life.

This is the story of how one neurotic, self-absorbed, occluded individual came, through his own personal experience, to realize the truth of the above paragraphs.

I suspect that there are many people like me who spend a great deal of their life in suffering. We are plagued with heavy feelings that rob us of life, of interest, of energy. We don't know how to get free of these feelings – in fact we don't even know what they really are. Sometimes life seems hopeless, desperate, joyless.

But I have found a way out, a way that leads to exuberance, aliveness, peace, and fulfillment. I feel extremely blessed in proceeding from feeling miserable most of the time to now, at age 73, feeling content most of the time. I am able to immensely appreciate the wonder and beauty around me, the joy of being with good friends, the marvelous sustenance and euphoria that comes from sharing deeply with my partner, and having a fulfilling sense of meaning and purpose in life. I am grateful to the many exceptional friends who have been so very supportive and helpful, and particularly for finding a path which kept me moving, though at times quite errantly, on the path to fuller realization.

• • •
• •
•

We are crossing northern Arizona on a mid-September morning, following Interstate 40. The year is 1990. My wife is driving, and I am sitting at my lap word processor, attempting to describe the state I am experiencing.

It is a real test of my writing ability, for how can mere words possibly convey the grandeur and the beauty we are immersed in? It is outstanding countryside, taking us first through canyons and rugged mountains, with marvelously sculpted rock formations, alive with a palette of colors. Each hill has its own distinctive surface, carved into gullies and walls that form its individual character, reflecting light and revealing shadows that make up a fascinating picture. The ridges rise one beyond the other, under the commanding surveillance of the highest peaks. Time is non-existent; the myriad manifestations of nature's most powerful forces demonstrate unending eras of time that make a single human lifetime a passing second. Yet the impact of the vast eras is very much in evidence, testimony to the wonder and mystery of the forces that shape the surface of our planet.

Further on, the landscape evolves to long-stretching, green plateaus, bounded by rising slopes of dark green, wooded hills. The fields are alive with flowers, countless brown-eyed Susans lining the highway, with a groundcover of tiny yellow daisies extending as far as the eye can reach. All under a pale cerulean sky, with just a few puffy, distinctively shaped clouds to add interest.

But all of this is only a hint of the penetrating sense of Presence that permeates it all. I can feel the radiant light that descends and suffuses everything, that sharpens the detail, and illuminates distinctive shapes and patterns of the vegetation, that gives a sense of wonder and some powerful, inexpressible meaning to everything in view. By simply sitting, observing, and appreciating, the light and underlying meaning grow in intensity, and I am filled with overflowing gratitude for the goodness, wonder, and beauty that our Creator has bestowed upon us.

I am not under the influence of any substance. But I am at a place that I have always longed to be, prayed to be, and for which I have undergone many years of intense searching and learning and finding, to finally taste the joy of communing even meagerly with the Divine Presence. And hopefully to learn more about how to stay in this communion.

I'm beginning to run out of feeling and am writing somewhat on memory. So I do what I've learned to do – become extremely still, quiet my mind, and allow space for God to reenter my awareness. Hopefully He will bring some inspiration.

How do you write of the Infinite? How do you describe the grandeur? How can you describe feelings that go beyond anything you have ever felt before? There must be new words for states of joy, states of ecstasy, states of fulfillment and satisfaction. Do they exist in Sanskrit? I am not enough of a scholar to know, but the Easterners have been exploring these states for many centuries, and no doubt have a much better vocabulary. They probably have not been translated into English, for in the objectively-oriented West there is little knowledge of the referents.

Now that I have opened myself up, waves of joy sweep over me and I am transfixed by the surrounding beauty – marvelous green meadows, flower-studded, with pine trees standing as guardians at the edges. The high mountains in the distance have a nostalgic appeal.

Now Mount Humphreys comes into view. It has the gentle slope of high volcanic mountains like those forming the island of Hawaii. Why have such mountains always moved me so? They are commanding; their towering height is indicative of great accomplishment and stature, they carry the scars of countless centuries of erosion and proudly wear the marks left by sun and rain and snow and freezing winds. But more than that, they are a symbol of greatness, of majesty, of the recognition of a superior order of things. I am reminded of the slogan carved across the top of a California government building in Sacramento: "Give me Men to Match my Mountains".

What a privilege to ride along in an automobile and look out on such beauty, to feel the marvelous sense of joy and Presence. I feel the forces of evolution; I can almost observe the course of developing civilizations.

But then I become aware of the pain and suffering of the world. And the profound sadness of realizing that a simple change of attitude on the part of people everywhere will resolve most of the difficulties. I am torn by the contrast between the misery of the world and the sublimity of my current connection to the Central Source of life and energy. I fervently wish that humans everywhere might have the privilege of experiencing this joy and this wisdom. The constant questions are: How may others experience this? Is there any way to help?

I hope my own life journey will yield some useful information for others seeking to answer the above two questions. My own search has been long and arduous. My primary interest has always been personal growth, another way of saying how to learn to feel good. Having a reasonably good analytical mind, I have always sought the most effective means. I believe that I have discovered what works best for me.

I am excited by the path of development I have followed, and I feel privileged to have experienced the things that have happened to me.

My path has been primarily that of psychedelic exploration. From my very first experience in April, 1956, I concluded that LSD is the most profound learning tool available to man. It took many years to become familiar with the characteristics and potential of this and similar substances, and with the most appropriate ways to use them. Many more years of study and application brought a steady increase in growth of awareness and knowledge. These substances are very powerful, and they give access to vast dimensions of the human mind for which we westerners have very little understanding. Used with little skill or knowledge, they can produce very unsettling experiences – so unsettling that the medical profession has chosen the term psychotomimetic (psychosis-mimicking) to describe them. What may be worse, they may produce convictions of new, superior wisdom without revealing how to employ such wisdom in ordinary life. Some are convinced they have the ultimate answers, yet are still unaware of their own self-deceptions. While very much at home in the levels of universal love and Oneness, they have failed to resolve deeply established habits that interfere with the expression of integrity and compassion in their day-to-day life.

But as way-showers of appropriate values and behavior and revealers of man's ultimate capabilities, they have in my opinion no equal anywhere. Best results are obtained when used in conjunction with an on-going spiritual discipline and practice, and in the companionship of experienced and knowledgeable associates. Prime prerequisites for these journeys are honesty and a true appreciation for life in all its bountifulness. Commitment to the welfare of oneself and others favorably enhances the outcome.

My experience with psychedelics, greatly enriched in the latter years of my life by exposure to some of the practices of Tibetan Buddhist meditation, has opened up extended areas of understanding. The famous Swiss psychiatrist Carl Jung has stated that realization of our ultimate self is a process of making the unconscious conscious. Psychedelic substances greatly facilitate this process. Jung has shown us through his relentless, fearless, dedicated exploration of his own unconscious that the unconscious reveals an enormous range of wisdom – from one's own hidden personal dynamics, to the archetypes underlying human behavior and development, and finally to the very essential nature of reality and creation.

A very important aspect of these inner dynamics is our Shadow. My own experience powerfully confirms Jung's emphasis on the importance of encountering and integrating shadow material. The Shadow, which includes all of the painful and undesirable material in our lives which we desperately wish to hide from consciousness, imprisons a great part of our energy and unconsciously exerts a powerful influence upon our behavior against our will. Yet it contains the energy and wisdom which will make us whole, give us true understanding and a real zest for life.

Shadow material is extremely difficult to face and acknowledge. The failure to do so, I am convinced, is largely responsible for the world's difficulties, and particularly the pain and suffering of the world. Lack of understanding of shadow material is responsible for our enormous drives of self-interest – for the greed, anger, and striving for status and domination that stands in the way of human compassion, harmony, true wisdom, and creativity.

Facing my own shadow has been enormously difficult and painful. I feel certain that I could never have approached it in any depth without the aid of psychedelic substances. These have helped in two ways. The first is through their wondrous ability to dissolve defenses and resistances for the earnest explorer, so that access to powerful unconscious material is permitted.

More important, they allow access to the Celestial level and the discovery of the Divine Love and Grace which permeate the universe. If one can reach this level of experience, it is so overpowering and leads to such utter gratitude and trust that there is no hesitation in putting oneself in the hands of the Supreme Teacher. One is willingly led, if need be, through the dungeons of human agony and the distortions of one's own personal creations to achieve freedom, understanding, and a more profound level of love.

I wish very much to share with you what has been a most exciting journey for me, a journey which has been wondrously fulfilling. The following pages summarize my life in the psychedelic world. It starts with my spiritual quest and introduction to what I prefer to call the sacraments. This led to the establishment of The International Foundation for Advanced Study in Meno Park, California, where research was conducted with LSD and mescaline for 3-1/2 years under the supervision of psychiatrist Charles Savage,

M.D. Another twenty years was spent researching promising new compounds as they became available.

Throughout this time, I was busily engaged in my own personal development process, which is documented in considerable detail as drug trials progressed. Because my marriage relationship was so central to my personal growth, I have devoted a separate chapter to provide an overview of this part of my life. I also report on experiments with other persons and with a variety of compounds.

To restrict interference with the flow of the narrative, I have compiled certain accumulations of data and conclusions in four Appendixes in the back, and refer to them in the text where appropriate. These appendixes may be consulted to clarify language or concepts used in the individual reports.

There is much confusion and misinformation in the world concerning psychoactive drugs, what they do, and their potential usefulness. Work reported here indicates a number of valuable applications, and considerable potential to enhance learning. All of this can be accomplished comfortably and safely with informed use. The potential value seems to clearly indicate the initiation of new scientific research in this field.

I hope that you will enjoy and find useful what follows.

# Chapter 1
# Early Beginnings

One afternoon some years ago I was discussing my resistance to writing with a good friend, an extraordinarily competent person. Despite having just gone through an earth-shaking experience, I couldn't mobilize the energy to write. There were years of accumulated data to digest, which seemed a heavy burden. And new information was constantly turning up.

He suggested, "Why not start in the middle? Make 'now' the middle, and go on from there".

There was something appealing about the idea – probably the freshness of the approach, since I tend to be stodgy and quite organized most of the time. Maybe the uniqueness of such a start would loosen some of the strands of creativity. But yet – I wasn't ready. There was still a major problem.

The experience just behind me was one of the most powerful of my life. But how would it turn out?

I have been blessed by many outstanding, profound experiences in my life. But there is something more important than having experiences, wonderful as they may be. I wished these marvelous states of realization to stay with me all the time. The trouble was, most of the time I found myself back in what Aldous Huxley called my "old stinking, sweating self." Not entirely; there was always some change. But not as much as I wanted. Would my enthusiasm over this last profound experience fade away as had the others?

Over the two months following this very special experience, a fascinating change began to evolve. I found more and more how to maintain the exalted state I had been seeking. It was so fulfilling that I knew I must begin to write.

This special event modified my whole approach to learning. To describe this occasion in an appropriate perspective, I wish to go back in time and retrace the events that led to this experience.

My spiritual awakening started around 1950, when I was 30 years old. It's difficult to focus on that time of my life without invoking the uncomfortable feelings I underwent almost continuously. I was extraordinarily neurotic, completely shut up within myself. I lived mostly inside my head, in fantasy. Extremely sensitive, I was self-conscious and uncomfortable most of the time. Many people were difficult to be around. I was so involved with myself that I hardly noticed others. Yet it was extremely important for me to have other people's acceptance, to the extent that I often found it difficult to express what I truly thought and felt in fear of incurring disfavor. So I repressed an enormous amount of anger. Because of my continual discomfort, I was constantly alert for any method to ease the pain.

I had a few good qualities. I was reasonably bright, having graduated first in my high school class and at the local military junior college in my home town of Roswell, New Mexico. At Stanford University, I was granted both a Phi Beta Kappa key and a Tau Beta Pi key in recognition of outstanding scholarship in both the arts and in engineering. I was also awarded a couple of fellowships which allowed me to take a year of graduate study in electrical engineering and get a master's degree.

One of my innate gifts, which I didn't recognize until recently, is an excellent sense of balance, of appropriateness, which has always allowed me to keep things in proper perspective. This helped lead to a successful career in industry. I had an excellent sense of the warranted time and energy each department should expend in accomplishing corporate objectives. I was also able to get members of different departments to understand each other and their functions, and how they could best work together to iron out operational difficulties.

My major vocational accomplishment was growing up with Ampex Corporation. Ampex started as a very small, obscure firm manufacturing electric motors and grew into a world leader in the field of magnetic recording. I progressed from design engineer of magnetic recording components to production engineer to application engineer to Director of Instrumentation Sales to Assistant to the President for Long Range Planning.

It was in the last position that I had my first encounter with LSD. At the time I was familiar with the frontiers of many technological fields of knowledge, for we were designing special magnetic recording equipment to aid research in most of those fields: telemetering essential information from missiles and aircraft that would aid in making design decisions, automotive engineering, geophysical exploration, recording the output of various sensing devices in laboratories, computers, and finally developing the world's first successful video tape recorder. I felt abreast of most scientific developments. Yet after my first LSD experience, I stated with confidence about LSD: "This is the greatest discovery that man has ever made." While I have learned a great deal in the ensuing years about proper use and misuse of this substance, nothing has ever brought into question the accuracy of this evaluation.[1]

There were several key events that led me to LSD. The first commenced one afternoon when I received a phone call from Clarence. Clarence was both a neighbor and a mechanical engineer at Ampex. He was a very quiet, likable, unassuming fellow whom I found it very easy to be with. We found we could very naturally discuss many areas involving depth of meaning not encountered in usual social conversations.

Clarence was going to a series of lectures, and he thought I would enjoy the speaker. It had been many years since I had attended a lecture. I was completely focused on work and contributing what I could to help a new, budding company get started and grow healthily. I felt ready for a change of pace. Since I trusted Clarence's judgment and liked being with him, I agreed to attend.

The lectures were held in a small library in South Palo Alto, just off the Stanford campus. The lecturer was Harry Rathbun, a professor of business law at Stanford University. Harry was a striking individual – tall, handsome, graying, with a remarkably saintly demeanor. Kindness and concern exuded from him. And he was a commanding speaker. I didn't find out until later that students at Stanford University had voted him a favorite among teachers. His last class of the year in business law, where he discussed personal ethics and values, overflowed with students coming from all over the school to hear his now-famous address.

His lectures hit me between the eyes. As he started, and warmed up to his topic, I found I was starved for the information he was imparting. After the first lecture, I could not possibly miss the remaining five. I didn't remember ever being as stimulated by a speaker. I hung on his every word.

The theme of his lectures was: Who are we? Where are we going? Are we still evolving? Do we have any evidence to answer these questions? I hadn't realized it, but I was deeply concerned about these topics. Perhaps the more so because I had pushed such considerations totally out of my life while I established a profession and a career in magnetic recording. I was as ready as hot sand in the desert for rainfall.

Harry convinced me of the enormity of human potential, of the necessity to wake up and take charge of our evolution, that we had a hallowed destiny, and that we could reach it by taking charge of our personal growth. I was thrilled by the picture that he painted.

Then he threw me a curve. In his last lecture, he addressed the means by which we could begin to accomplish this splendid goal. It was by studying the teachings of Jesus!

As a Jew, I felt I had been led down a garden path. What a sneaky trap! I was infuriated. Yet I had been deeply touched. So the following year, when Harry Rathbun led a series of discussion groups, I was drawn to them once more. When I set aside my bias against Jesus and my feelings about what has happened to Jews around the world in his name, I found what was proposed very much to my liking. We followed a text *Jesus as Teacher* by Henry Burton Sharman.[2] The author had spent thirty years critically examining biblical texts, extracting what he believed to be the essence of Jesus's teachings. We examined this book with a hard-headed, down-to-earth approach to answer the questions: Do his teachings make any sense? Has he found any truth? Is there any value there for us as individuals in leading our personal lives?

I found I very much enjoyed participating in this examination, and joined a discussion group. I liked working in the group, the friendships that arose, the challenge of the material, and the answers that began to emerge with ever-growing clarity and power. A two-week seminar led by Harry Rathbun and his wife Emilia greatly intensified our search and discussions. By the time the seminar was over, I experienced true love for others for the first time in my life, and became convinced of the power of the message of Jesus. When his teachings were separated from the frills, beliefs, and projections, the impact was enormous. I was inescapably led to the conclusion that the most important thing I can do with my life is to commit myself to the will of God. A great deal of the discussion focused on what this meant and how to do it.

It was while attending this seminar that I had my first real mystical experience. One evening, lying on the floor of the lodge where we met, I was looking up through the glass skylight at the redwood trees beautifully illuminated by moonlight, listening to Gregorian chants. I suddenly felt a pain in my chest – a deep, profound feeling that was ecstatic despite the pain. Never before had I encountered such a feeling. It was from another dimension. I knew with absolute conviction that I was being touched by God.

Previously I had been willing to believe in God, but my belief was speculation. Now I was convinced that God was real, and that I could experience His very Presence!

I was enormously moved by the impact of this discovery. I started getting up every morning to meditate, and my experiences immediately became intense and insightful. At the same time, I began reading every important book on psychology and mysticism that I could get my hands on.

It is no wonder, then, that I joined this group and became an active member. I served several years on the planning committee, which comprised the most dedicated of the followers. We not only served as a management advisory council for the organization known as the Sequoia Seminar, but conducted many activities for our own self-growth.

I might be with them yet, if another powerfully influential figure had not strolled into my life.

I have been most fortunate in meeting several outstanding people in my life. Gerald Heard was certainly one of them. My first encounter with him was hearing him lecture. Gerald was a good personal friend of Harry and Emelia Rathbun, the leaders of the Sequoia Seminar with whom I was deeply involved at the time. Gerald was probably one of the world's outstanding contemporary mystics, and was responsible for personally introducing Aldous Huxley to Eastern thought. This exposure made such a profound impression on Huxley that it completely altered the direction of his writing.

Gerald was a prolific writer himself, and wrote with great insight on humankind's evolutionary and spiritual development. One of his books, *Preface to Prayer*, made an enormous impact on me, opening my eyes to the possibility of other levels of reality beyond my usual engineering-focused concepts. Gerald also wrote very meaningfully on the subject of contemplative prayer, such as *Training for the Life of the Spirit.* Such works further reinforced my confidence in the reality of mystical levels of experience.

But what really struck me about Gerald was his power as a speaker. Although slight of build, he had a commanding voice and appearance. With his thoughtful face and handsome beard, he looked like a sage, and the beautiful flow of words that came from him proved that he was. In perfect diction, extraordinarily expressive prose, and with the accent and voice of authority that only an Englishman can muster, his words came across forming beautiful images and profound stirrings of understanding. Gerald specialized in conceptual thinking, so that he was a master of tying together various elements of human exploration and understanding to form higher and higher levels of significance. I found listening to him to be truly transporting.

I was so impressed with Gerald that I went to visit him in Pacific Palisades whenever my company business took me to Los Angeles, which was rather frequently. So when Gerald led a two-week seminar at the Sequoia

Seminar lodge, I was delighted to attend. It was a dynamic, growth-stimulating, inspiring seminar. This image that I have retained through the years perhaps best gives the flavor of it:

Gerald would come into the meeting room, which was hexagonal in shape, with windows all around giving excellent views of the surrounding hills and redwood trees. The group of some twenty persons sat opposite him as he took his chair near the center. He always came in with a huge sheaf of papers which he placed in his lap. He would then start his discourse, and for two hours he would flow like a fountain, his statements perfectly arranged, in exquisitely composed poetic prose. He spoke mostly of spiritual growth and development. An outstanding scholar, he was familiar with most of the works in the spiritual literature. He would quote names and dates, and often whole stanzas of poetry, without once looking at the papers he brought with him. It was as though his hand resting on the manila folder holding his papers made sufficient contact to draw up all the wisdom they contained.

An example of his creativity and the extreme fluidity of his mind came in an evening gathering. At dinner, one of the more aggressive and humorous members of our group said, "Gerald, why don't you spice things up a bit tonight and talk about SEX?" Everyone, including Gerald, laughed.

That evening, at every opportunity, he wove into the fabric of his discourse anecdotes regarding women in the early history of the church. He covered the trials and tribulations of the sexes attempting to relate, especially in regard to celibacy and the difficulties of maintaining it in the interest of spiritual growth. His penetrating insight and good humor kept us all laughing.

One evening when I was visiting Gerald in his home in Pacific Palisades, he went on at length about the outstanding virtues of LSD. I could hardly believe him; I could not understand why a person of his gifts who could freely explore the cosmos with his mind would want to take a drug. He gave me excellent assurance of the value of this approach in a letter, and gave me the name of that strange Canadian who came down and sometimes administered LSD to him and Aldous Huxley. The man was Al Hubbard.

Hubbard didn't often cross my mind until Alexander Poniatoff, the Chairman of the Board of Ampex, with whom I was intimately related for a number of years, told me of meeting this fabulous character in Canada. The stories Al related concerning people he had cured using LSD were quite outlandish. This second exposure to Hubbard piqued my interest, and I wrote a long letter to Al concerning my spiritual aspirations and requesting more information about LSD. My letter must have impressed him, as it wasn't long until Al Hubbard called on me in person at Ampex.

Hubbard made a deeper impression on me than anyone I had ever met. It was an impression that radically altered my whole value-belief system, and completely changed the course of my life.

Hubbard ran into psychedelics in the early 1950's, when he became a research subject for experiments employing mescaline at the University of Vancouver. With his great sensitivity and free, intuitive mind, Al readily achieved remarkable experiences of mystical levels and enormous depths of understanding. Fully aware of the potential of such experiences, he used his very appreciable entrepreneurial abilities to acquire copious supplies of LSD.

Al developed what came to be know as "the overwhelming dose technique," discussed in Stanislov Grof's book *LSD Psychotherapy*[3] under the heading Psychedelic Therapy. He experimented widely, and reported excellent results in treating alcoholics and helping many others with serious emotional problems. He won the support of psychiatrists Humphry Osmond and Abram Hoffer in Saskatchewan by demonstrating that LSD was not a psychotomimetic as designated by the medical profession. Hubbard was able to help them set up appropriate methods employing LSD to treat alcoholism. With his outstanding success, he dedicated himself to teaching others how to employ this new tool. His enterprise ultimately led him to my office at Ampex.

What a contrast between he and me! Here I was, slight of build, deadly serious, extremely introverted, trembling at whether others approved of me or not, anxious to follow all the rules and conventions of society. And here was he, large in body, constantly grinning, with a mischievous twinkle in his eye, turning everything into fun. He was voracious in his appetites for all that life had to offer, and a great belittler of all that ordinary persons held dear. What a combination – my staid character that didn't wish to tread on anyone's toes, and he, constantly looking how to upset the status quo and produce some excitement.

Hubbard was warm and engaging, and a great story teller. There was so little warmth in my own life that I was rapidly roped in. And he was an expert in discerning one's weaknesses, and playing upon them to advantage. Which meant that he could be most appealing and charming if his aim was to build a friendship.

He had powerful tools to reinforce his own canniness. That first day, he took me to a motel where he and his wife and another traveling companion, a close friend of the family, were staying. He gave me a tablet of methedrine, which I had never before had, and then introduced me to Meduna's mixture of 70% oxygen and 30% carbon dioxide.[4] No doubt reading me quite accurately, he gave me only a few breaths, but it was enough to give me a glimpse, and especially a feeling, of another world. The contact was magical, and was retained and reinforced through the remainder of the day by the methedrine I had ingested. Never before had I felt such euphoria. And with his exciting stories, I was completely convinced that I had to try LSD.

Taking LSD with Hubbard meant going to Canada. Our first meeting had occurred in February, and Al wanted me to wait until spring when we could go to his island, a beautiful 28 acre wooded stretch of land in the Vancouver Gulf. However, I was too impatient, so he consented to let me come in April, and I had my first LSD experience in his apartment, April 12, 1956.

By the time I undertook this experience, I had talked at length with Al and had read a number of reports. I had no trouble accepting that our minds are infinite, that the total memories of our life are stored in and available in our unconscious, that our inner being is eternal and through it we can explore past lives, the evolution of our planet and our universe, and understand the workings of the cosmos. I was eager to verify these things for myself.

I was prepared for the experience by taking some additional inhalations of the Meduna 30-70 mixture, and on the morning of my experience, was introduced to Monsignor Brown, archbishop of the local Catholic Diocese. Father Brown gave his blessing for my journey and promised to remember me at noon Mass, when I would be in the heart of my venture.

I was given about 66 micrograms of LSD procured from the original manufacturer, Sandoz Pharmaceuticals. Al, his wife Rita, and an associate of Al's in this work, Bill Galleon, were my guides who supported me through this experience. The following are excerpts from my notes made a few days following the experience:

> I am very taken by the beauty of the music, a requiem. I have images of Catholic Priests preaching, exhorting their followers. I find it utterly hilarious, because they are so serious and don't have a clue as to what it is really all about. They talk about God but really know nothing of God. I laugh and laugh until my belly muscles are sore. I am told by my guides that this is the laughter I have suppressed in my life.
>
> Later in the experience I expect to journey back in time, similar to reports I had read, and look at the dinosaurs. Nothing like that is happening, and I am getting more and more uncomfortable. I am shown a picture of Christ, Veronica's Veil. The picture is designed so that one can see the eyes either open or shut. Jesus looks right at me, first with eyes open, then with eyes shut, then alternating. Suddenly the face changes completely! It is a female face! I look again closely, startled. As I look, another face swishes into its place, then another one. Suddenly the faces begin to change at an enormous rate, so that hundreds of faces sweep past me. Each one is crystal clear, complete in every detail. I see men, women, and children in all walks of life. I particularly remember a rabbi with a long flowing beard, a gruesome looking pirate with a black patch over one eye, a Chinaman with a long ponytail. The last two I somehow associate with Al. Finally it dawns on me. I say out loud, "This is every man."
>
> This is a shaking revelation. It brings complete relief from my feelings of discomfort. However they soon return and intensify. I lie down for two miserable hours, feeling I should relive my birth as others had done. I am unable to do so. Finally I am asked to sit up in a chair. This feels somewhat better. Bill asks, "Myron, who's approval did you seek?"
>
> I begin to think. Was it my father? I am able to run back through my life at a rapid pace, like rapidly turning pages in a book. I had perhaps picked this up from reading a report of Bill's. I can see and know with surety that it wasn't my father. I repeat the procedure with my mother. As I am doing this, I am suddenly caught in a horribly painful stance. My head is bent over, my body is under enormous pressure, the vertebrae in my back are crushed together as though being squeezed in a vise. The pain is unbearably excruciating. I feel I simply can't stand it. Suddenly I am propelled forward, and I am exploded from the birth canal!
>
> Several dramatic things happen simultaneously. First, the enormous release from the pain. Next, I feel as though I am suddenly struck by lightning, as an enormous burst of energy pervades my body. This is the release of a monumental charge of anger and an incredibly profound feeling of absolute worthlessness. I blurt out loud, "They couldn't wait for me to be born!!" And I can see doctors

> and nurses standing around while I smell the odor of ether just as clearly as if an ether-soaked wad of cotton were held right under my nose.
>
> I am shaken to the core. I can't believe that such an enormous charge of feeling had all this time been held below the surface of consciousness without my having a clue of its presence or content. I realize that I had been hung up in the process of being born, and had been under enormous pressure and pain for some time. I was no doubt causing my mother a lot of pain, and I felt utterly worthless and condemned for holding up the process and creating so much pain.
>
> At the same time I can rapidly scan my life and see how this had been the most powerful personality-forming dynamic. I can see how it affected my feelings, my responses, my entire way of conducting myself. It accounts for my deep sense of worthlessness, my drive for status and accomplishment, my intense eagerness to please others, my compulsion for never being late to an appointment. Enormous relief floods over me.
>
> This experience relieves the powerful uncomfortable feelings, and the remainder of the session is more enjoyable. I feel led through several interesting instructional experiences. At one point I am searching for God's will. Intense fear and tensions build up in my body, and it becomes clear that I must die. I put myself in a state of willingness, and then the tensions and fear suddenly lift. An inner voice says to me, "You only have to be *willing* to die; you don't actually have to die."

The impact that this experience had on me was enormous. We talk about the unconscious, and think we know what it is. But to suddenly be confronted with powerful unconscious material, to know that the unconscious is *really real*, to realize the utter power of it and not to have so much as a clue as to the root or nature of it!!

And the revelations also included profound realizations that God is absolutely real, and that there is only One Person, of which we are all a part. I held LSD to be the most important discovery man has ever made, and would devote my life to learning more about it and how to use it effectively, not only for myself but for others.

The next few years were spent in a number of exploratory avenues. There was no question that I was a zealot. I saw experiences like mine bringing answers to all of the world's problems, and providing humankind with the powerful tools needed for growth and development. There was much to learn. Who would be adequate subjects for this kind of exploration? How successful would such experiences be with different kinds of individuals? What would be the best procedures for utilizing such a powerful and outstanding tool?

First I went to my close associates in the Sequoia Seminar. While some of them had interesting and worthwhile experiences with LSD, they didn't particularly care for my now bosom buddy, Al Hubbard. They saw him as an enormous egotist; they were repulsed by his fun-loving manner which made light of their serious approach to life.

We formed an LSD research group, but there was dissension among the members. Each had a different plan, and was ready to substitute his/her personal speculations for Hubbard's extensive experience. To me, none of the plans showed promise compared to Hubbard's direct approach with proven results. So I moved out on my own.

I had been leading a Sequoia Seminar type discussion group for a couple of years, and was very close to all the members of the group. They decided to try LSD. One Monday night a member of the group would take LSD, and the rest of us would support her or him. The following Monday night the subject would share in detail his/her experience, and the following week we would proceed to the next member. All of the experiences were fruitful and valuable. We began to see differences in the responses of individuals, and the fact that there was a great variety of response, varying from psychological dynamics to mystical realizations.

I grew confident in my understanding of how to work with this substance, and verified that LSD was not a psychotomimetic as the medical profession claimed. I also understood why they made the claim. I see two major factors. If one has no understanding of the vast dimensions of the mind beyond ordinary experience (such as extra-sensory perception) or of the spiritual basis of reality, one might feel that experiencing such actualities is insanity.

The second factor involves the manner in which the experience is accepted. We found the action of the drug often worked to dissolve powerfully held false beliefs or painfully repressed or frightening feelings. This action often met with powerful resistance on the part of the subject. Surrendering to such experiences led to profound new understanding. Determined resistance, however, led to much pain and suffering, and sometimes escape into psychotic-type episodes. To avoid such discomfort, it is extremely important to approach psychedelic substances with good motivation, openness, and with a sincere desire to learn.

In the LSD state, it is possible to reach levels where the mind is sharp and clear. Fresh ideas and perspectives flow unhindered, presenting many new possibilities, often of great value. I felt that such heightened perceptions could be valuable in improving business operations. So I began to search for ways to utilize LSD at Ampex Corporation. At this time, I was Assistant to the President in Charge of Long Range Planning, and was a member of the Ampex Management Committee that reviewed and often arrived at management decisions for the Corporation. I made my proposal to the group, and immediately encountered enormous resistance. There was great fear of trying unknown substances on as delicate an organ as the brain. My own experience and that of Hubbard were completely discounted. I was too naive to understand why. So I went ahead on my own, selecting a group of engineers who were good friends and interested in the experiment. With the help of Hubbard and a physician friend, eight subjects underwent the experience at a cabin in the Sierra Nevada Mountains. There was a wide range of experiences, but all were impressed with the enormous openings of the mind, the ability to experience new levels of thought and comprehension, the gain in self-knowledge, and in some cases, the ability to solve technical problems. But much to my amazement, the results were totally ignored by management. I was to learn later that a member of our Board of Directors was also on the Board of the Palo Alto Research Center. He was strongly advised by the latter group to completely discourage me from this work, as I had no medical or therapeutic training.

My experience continued to grow, and I was awed at the ability to learn of mental processes well beyond my previous understanding. I also began to understood the enormous fear most persons had of psychedelic substances. Almost everyone has an innate fear of encountering the unconscious, as the unconscious mind contains much material that we wish to hide from ourselves. The fear and discomfort is often greater for professionals, who place great store on their special training. They cannot be sure how their values and functioning will appear in the light of cosmic truth. Dr. Abram Hoffer in Canada, who worked with LSD in the 1950s, found that ministers, psychologists, and psychiatrists often had the most uncomfortable experiences.

A key experience came for me in 1959, when I took a much larger dose than usual, 150 micrograms, Al deeming that I was ready for it. The outstanding event of this experience was a dramatic breakthrough in which I was shown that Jesus was God, and that *I* was God! With this realization I broke down completely and sobbed and sobbed without letup for fifteen minutes. Later I sat down to play the piano, and played as I have never played before. I felt that I was playing the music as the composer realized it, and able to express the marvelous depth of feeling the composer was portraying. This experience led to a quantum-step improvement in my ability to play the piano, which remained with me from that time on.

I had now gathered enough understanding that it was imperative to spend full time at this research. In 1961 I resigned from Ampex, set up a non-profit corporation which I boldly and naively named the International Foundation for Advanced Study, and located offices and research space in the town of Menlo Park, California, where I lived. I was encouraged in this step by several good friends familiar with the potential of psychedelics, and who later joined the staff of the Foundation.

With the help of Al Hubbard, we succeeded in obtaining Charles Savage as our Medical Director. Dr. Savage was a psychiatrist who had done some research with psychedelic materials, and looked forward to doing more work in this field.

Over the next 3-1/2 years, some 350 clients were processed through the program at the Foundation. A great deal was discovered about the effective use of these substances and the enormous potential they offer for numerous avenues of research. Dr. Savage assembled a number of volunteers to be part of the research staff which planned and gathered important elements of information. We learned many important principles for conducting psychedelic sessions, selecting subjects, responses to expect, and the follow-up that was required.

An early lesson was the disadvantage of treating only one member of an unhappy marriage. The experience often widened the rift between the couple. We established the policy of requiring both parties to participate. An exception was the case where the untreated party was deemed mature and thoroughly supported the partner through the psychedelic experience and the outcome.

One of our therapists, Don Allen, was a former Ampex engineer. Because of his and my background, we attracted a number of engineers to our program. We found engineers often to be unusually sensitive individuals. Because of their sensitivity, they found many of their early life experiences painful. This resulted in the choice of a vocation that dealt with inanimate objects, sparing further emotional pain. LSD was a marvelous tool for discovering and releasing buried feelings. Through such discoveries, many engineers found the importance of feelings of love and intimacy. These subjects gained substantially in their ability to express feelings and avoid pain through appropriate communication. The result was significant improvement in their marriage relationships and in dealing with their children.

Great gains were made by most subjects in understanding their personal dynamics, improving relationships and communication, improving their ability to function in the workplace, and achieving an enhanced sense of well-being. Many reached rewarding levels of spiritual realization, recognizing the harmony and oneness of life, and the power of love to resolve problems and conflicts.

About one half those treated for alcoholism stopped drinking after a single LSD experience. Even with those not cured, there were some salutary effects. One alcoholic subject declared our treatment a failure, as he started drinking again within a week. "Alcoholics Anonymous was the real cure," he told me. Before he came to us, he had staunchly refused any contact with AA.

We used several instruments to assess change as a result of undergoing a psychedelic experience in the Foundation program. The most definitive results came from the use of a test called the MMPI, or Multiphasic Personality Inventory. This test is commonly used by psychologists to assess personality patterns. It is "well-constructed, empirically-derived, and extensively validated." (See Appendix I, Mogar and Savage, 1964.) Typical scales of assessment are ego strength, anxiety, repression, rigidity, prejudice, ego overcontrol, neurotic over- and under-control, and evaluation of improvement.

Robert Mogar, Ph.D., Associate Professor of Psychology at San Francisco State College, had a great deal of experience in assessing the results obtained with the MMPI. Robert joined the Foundation research staff to aid in assessing changes in subjects undergoing the psychedelic experience. Participants were tested with the MMPI before their experience, two months after, and six months after their experience.

In the historical use of the MMPI to assess improvement in various kinds of therapy, studies have reported slight or unreliable changes, or at best slight but significant changes only in cases that were judged clinically improved. One investigator had judged that the MMPI must be insensitive to improvement, since the findings were consistently negative.

Much to Robert's surprise, as he compared tests before and after the LSD experience, there were significant shifts in scales, even those held by the profession to be fairly stable. He reported that these shifts were greater than any he had previously seen. All groups tested showed significant improvement over the pre-treatment test at the two month mark. While the most disturbed group showed some regression to their previous state at the six months test, they were still improved at this time. The improvement for the more moderate groups held up quite well at six months. These results were obtained on subjects who had undergone only a single psychedelic experience.

A detailed description of the results using the MMPI evaluations is given in the paper Mogar and Savage, 1964, Appendix I. Other aspects of the studies conducted by the Foundation research staff have been published in appropriate medical journals. These papers are listed in Appendix I.

I must comment, however, on an aspect of the work that never failed to impress me. Each morning I would come to work and park in the Menlo Park downtown parking lot which adjoined our building. As I looked up at the suite of offices that had been especially designed to conduct our work (and which resided over a beauty parlor!), I could not help but be awed at the enormous contrast between what was taking place in these offices and the understanding of the people parking in the lot below. Twice a week, two or more individuals were exploring ranges of perception and understanding beyond the comprehension of most persons in our society. Those doing their downtown shopping had no idea of what transpired in these offices.

In industry, if one should be so fortunate as to advance the state of the art with some new discovery, it is usually only a matter of months – at most a year or two – before competitors find a solution and offer the same development. But despite the important new knowledge being revealed regarding the human mind, there was little curiosity in our work.

I had another extremely important personal experience during this time. The circumstances were indeed odd.

Back in those days, the very thought of encountering my unconscious and levels of truth would fill me with profound anxiety. But this time the circumstances were simple. My good friend Al sent me down an ampoule of LSD that had been put up by another chemical firm, and asked me to try it to see how it compared to that manufactured by Sandoz. So I flew to the desert with our good friend Jerome.

Jerome was a very large, good-looking, very personable fellow. He was great fun to be with, but a bit unscrupulous in his dealings in used machinery. He and Al had a lot in common and made a great pair. Jerome agreed to fly me over, and we drove to Death Valley in the 1962 Impala I kept at the desert airport.

Since my goal was simply to evaluate the activity of the new ampoule, I was under no pressure to solve problems or deal with uncomfortable feelings. I imbibed in the sands of the Valley floor, and when I felt the effect, Jerome drove me back to Lone Pine. Here is what happened:

> We had hardly started our drive back when I looked up at the sky above the surrounding hills, and a powerful biblical phrase hit me. I am today unable to remember the words, but the effect on me was utterly profound. Suddenly I realized that I was God! Everything opened up. I cast off my body like a shell, and was totally free! The freedom was combined with an outstanding euphoria.
>
> But most important of all was the wisdom. I felt as though I *knew everything*, and only had to turn my attention to the subject to see it clearly. First I saw deeply into the meaning of life. It was a beautiful dance, and I could see it portrayed in the heavens. I saw a small figure, which represented our little self,

> pursuing a giant figure, which is our Real Self. This is the dance of life and the purpose of life, for the little self to catch and join and realize the Real Self, the most fulfilling and joyous thing that can possibly happen. All the joy, all the sorrow, all the delight, all the pain and suffering were merely aspects of this wonderful dance. The crowning of all fulfillment is the achievement of this most magnificent Union when the little self merges with the Real Self. And when this happened to me, I found that I am truly God. I am part and parcel of the whole universe, and had created it all. I only needed to look and see how I had done it.
>
> We passed the desert floor of Panamint Valley, where many rocks were strewn across the valley floor. I saw them piled up as human skulls, thousands upon thousands of them piled up in stacks. These were the skulls of those who had died without finding me. I wept for sadness. But as soon as I wept, flowers sprang up all over the world.

For days I was walking on air. But the exuberance of this state departed, and once more I was back, as Aldous Huxley has described, in "my old stinking self." However, I could never forget the true significance of it, and would forever address myself to achieving this state on a more enduring basis. It would take a number of years to discover the requirements to reach and maintain this state.

As the work of the Foundation progressed, there were a few professional foundations who became interested in what we were doing, and we received some invitations to apply for grants for specific kinds of research. However, with the advent of Timothy Leary and the enormous adverse publicity created by his activities, the scientific interest in this field evaporated. At one point, San Francisco State College responded favorably to the request of members of our Foundation staff to set up a new Institute specifically for psychedelic research. But as the rumble of unfavorable publicity raised to a roar, they no longer wished to be associated with it.

In 1965, Dr. James Goddard was appointed the new director of the FDA. He brought a halt to all LSD research in the nation that was involved with humans and the exploration of consciousness. This terminated the work of the Foundation. We subsisted another year while we submitted a new IND for the use of mescaline, but ultimately this too was denied (the letters IND stand for Investigational New Drug exemption, which is the authorization that permits research to be conducted on new drugs that have not yet been approved by the FDA). Fortunately it permitted sufficient time to do our creativity study, which is considered by many to be an important addition to the body of literature on psychedelic research.[5]

So the Foundation was closed and professional interest in psychedelics lapsed into disfavor. The key psychedelics were placed in Schedule 1 of the Controlled Substances Act of 1970.[6]

The net result of these developments was that no legitimate research was conducted with psychedelic substances for over two decades. All those interested in such compounds have been driven underground, so that the outcome of such work remains generally unknown to the public and other researchers.

The closing of the Foundation was a very crippling blow to me. It was hard to accept a world that rejected research that offered so much promise for the general welfare. It was extremely difficult to turn away from activities which were revealing solutions to humanity's most pressing problems and deepest needs.

My wounds slowly healed and I adjusted to a much more ordinary life. This included divorcing my first wife, getting remarried, and reconciling to a new wife and an adopted eleven year old daughter. It also included finding a comfortable position in industry. My new occupation was managing a small firm that produced sound filmstrips for use in the social studies curriculum of secondary schools.

It would be several years before a new door opened, which would allow me to once more pursue my major interest.

**Chapter 1 Notes**

1. My logic is as follows: The most important thing in the universe is Mind, which is infinite and all-comprehensive, and reveals to man his total nature. While many aspects of mind have been discovered by adepts through the ages, including the complete enlightenment of the Buddha, LSD offers the serious, dedicated seeker who searches with integrity access to aspects and levels of mind beyond any other practice or aid of which I know. The only ones who would argue with this conclusion are so adept in their practice that their experience is considerably beyond the grasp of the vast majority of the world's population.
2. Sharman, H. B. *Jesus as Teacher*. New York and London: Harper and Brothers, 1935.
3. Grof, S. *LSD Psychotherapy*. Pomona, California: Hunter House, 1980, pp. 32-37.
4. Meduna, L. J. *Carbon Dioxide Therapy*. Springfield, Ill.: Charles C. Thomas, 1950. Meduna discovered that inhaling a mixture of 70% oxygen and 30% carbon dioxide provided an experience of an altered state of consciousness, often accompanied by substantial abreaction. With proper preparation and administration, he found that clients could be helped considerably to become free of their neuroses.

   Inhaling a sufficient number of breaths of this mixture has the effect of dissolving the resistances holding down repressed feelings, permitting their expression. There is usually a rapid succession of imagery, and the discharge of feelings is often accompanied by a considerable amount of insight. In our Foundation work with clients, we found that several treatments with this mixture was an excellent procedure to introduce novices to altered states of consciousness. Many discovered unconscious contents of their mind for the first time. The procedure also cleared away a good deal of repressed material, thus freeing the subject for a smoother, more profound psychedelic experience.
5. Harman, W. W., McKim, R. H., Mogar, R. E., Fadiman, J., and Stolaroff, M. "Psychedelic Agents in Creative Problem-Solving: A Pilot Study." *Psychological Reports* 19: 211-227, 1966.
6. The requirements for a substance to be placed in Schedule I are as follows:

   (A). The drug or other substance has a high potential for abuse.

   (B). The drug or other substance has no currently accepted medical use in treatment in the United States.

   (C). There is a lack of accepted safety for use of the drug or other substance under medical supervision.

   Schedule 1 items are illegal to possess, and from a practical standpoint it has been impossible to conduct research with them. While there are provisions for conducting research with Schedule I materials, they are so complex and stringent that most researchers prefer to work in other areas. Research with Schedule I materials also requires that the FDA approve the research protocol, and for many years it has been extremely difficult to obtain such approval for psychedelic-type materials. Review boards for research protocols are generally chosen from well-known experts in the field being investigated. In the case of psychedelics this has not been the case. The members of the medical community chosen to sit in judgement on these protocols seldom have had first-hand knowledge and experience with such substances and have not been favorable to allowing research to proceed.

In recent times, a more receptive attitude has been demonstrated both by the FDA and NIDA, the National Institute of Drug Abuse. They have announced a willingness to consider carefully prepared protocols for psychedelic research, and hopefully some projects may soon be started.

What is required are qualified researchers who are sufficiently committed to the process to design satisfactory projects and patiently shepherd them through the various steps required to obtain the IND which authorizes such research to be conducted. It may also require considerable effort to round up the necessary funds to support the work.

# Chapter 2
# The Interim Years

In time, I put the closing of the Foundation behind me and accommodated to my new circumstances. The difficulties of adjusting were eased by continuing my own private investigations into the use of that exceptional mind-opening substance, LSD.

After a time I began to notice a pattern in my experiences. The first few hours were very uncomfortable. Everything that was wrong with me was readily apparent. I felt worthless, and that everything I was doing was wrong. The feelings were miserable. I would work through these feelings and begin to feel better. Then my mind would clear up and I would begin to put things in perspective. The miserable feelings would depart and I would be filled with love. My consciousness would then rise to clearer perception, and I would begin to think in larger frames of reference. At this level I not only had a clear view of my personal functioning and relationships, but I could also perceive the evolution and dynamics of society. I could recognize social problems and their solutions. Most clear was the importance of having an intimate relationship with the Supreme Teacher.

At the end of the experience I would feel euphoric and revitalized, and feel this way for one to two weeks. Then I would begin to feel bogged down again and wish to have another experience to achieve clarity.

There was always some learning and improvement, and life steadily got better. I was also considerably expanding my understanding of human dynamics, the nature of the psyche, and the spiritual levels of reality. Despite my on-going relapses into negative states, the grip of such feelings lessened and my overall state of being improved.

I was delighted that Jean, whom I married in 1970, loved to share psychedelic experiences. Jean accepted life more gracefully than I, and consequently was not as interested as I was to discover new modes of functioning. Our relationship was the central element of most of our explorations and focus on growth. The history of this relationship is detailed in Chapter 14, Story of a Marriage.

I noticed that in attending retreats or conferences with other people engaged in the spiritual search, the others were often struggling with issues that had cleared up for Jean and me through psychedelic exploration. Also, we had ceased to fuss about the distractions and irritations in life and relationships which still preoccupied many of the others.

But it took a long time for me to eradicate the powerful negative feelings that often erupted. I found it necessary to go deeply into myself to learn the real source of my ongoing discomfort, and how to resolve it. It is only in recent times that I feel that what I have learned has been integrated into real wisdom, with accompanying ongoing well-being.

Change is very difficult, and it took me a long time to realize that in many respects I was not changing, but simply relying on further experiences for well-being. But despite my stubbornness and unwillingness to change, insights did impress themselves upon me, and some change came about.

The year 1978 brought on a new era. An old friend looked me up. He wondered how my investigations were proceeding. When I replied that the law had terminated such work, he was surprised (the Controlled Substances Act of 1970 made all of the major psychedelics illegal to possess). He told me that there was a great number of new substances that were not scheduled (not placed in Schedule I of the Controlled Substances Act, the schedule that carries the most severe restrictions and penalties).

This opened a new door for which I was immensely grateful. For the next several years, my wife and I became familiar with a number of new compounds. With the most promising ones, we extended our investigations to a number of other people to learn more completely the nature of these substances, compare them with the older, scheduled ones, and determine if they were generally useful without hindering side-effects.

It was during these endeavors that I had another life-changing, breakthrough experience. This is the one that inspired the process of recording my adventures, referred to at the beginning of Chapter 1. It was a most significant personal experience that profoundly a ffected my conduct of this research and substantially improved my rate of growth:

> This was my first experience of a very powerful substance, DOET, and was taken in a group. I started with a moderate dose of 2 m.g., but before long I felt that the amount of repressed psychic material that needed processing would require a greater dose, so I took an additional 2 m.g. at the two hour point.
>
> It was a strange day. I alternated between entering sublime spaces, and regressing into hostile, infantile states. My mood grew blacker as the day progressed. This substance was extremely long acting. By bedtime I was very tired but still very hyper and agitated. It was a relief to crawl into bed, snuggle up to Jean, and release to the experience.
>
> I turned my attention inside and surrendered to the experience. Relief came promptly with marvelous visuals – beautiful plastic materials and liquids, exquisite blues and other intense colors. It soon came to me that the most important thing was to TRUST. I turned over my trust to whatever wished to happen. I would find myself approaching an abyss that seemed terribly frightening. Yet when I gave my trust to the process, an important, meaningful experience developed, dissipating the discomfort and resulting in a growing feeling of aliveness.
>
> It soon became apparent that there was a magnificent, beneficent force behind this whole process, and the best thing I could possibly do was turn myself over completely to this wonderful energy. As I did, it led to noteworthy experiences and realizations. I felt I was surrendering myself to Myself, the central, all-wise, all-knowing teacher, totally concerned with my well-being. As tension built up, which occurred after each release, it would be dissipated with the understanding of what caused it and how to be free of it.
>
> It became clear that my need to be right and my fear of making mistakes were severe blocks to proper functioning. As I relinquished these fixations, I became more relaxed. As the process continued, inappropriate behavior patterns came into view, and I could drop them like deleting files on a computer. I would immediately feel increased energy, aliveness, and well-being. I dropped defensiveness; I realized that changes didn't happen immediately but took time.

It's all right to be uncomfortable – just trust what is. A great deal of my difficulty stemmed from straining to make things different than they are. I simply need to trust and stop using so much energy. What is truly appropriate can be found by looking deeply within myself.

For several years I had been suffering from prostatitis, which made urinating difficult and irritating. Thinking about my prostate problem, I felt the enormous fear of undergoing surgery. I saw this was linked to the injury and injustice I had felt from adenoids and other operations in my early childhood. If surgery was necessary, I could simply trust my way through it. I was able to see that the medical people in my childhood were doing their best to help me and that I could trust them.

A marvelous realization came over me. All normal body functions feel good. For several years it has been uncomfortable to urinate, a procedure which should feel quite good and bring a wonderful sense of relief. It seemed that my prostate and urinary problem stemmed from the way that I was distorting life. I was dying, withdrawing from life. I see that I must vote for life – let the old structures drop away and focus on and make way for the new. This way new life and new energy can manifest. Just realizing this seemed to wipe away huge sets of programs in my being. This brought a gratifying sense of renewal and a discerning appreciation of my body and its functions.

As I confronted each uncomfortable feeling and turned it over to Trust, I became more free and ecstatic. I realized that the Self who is my Teacher is the only reality that is important. The intimacy and communication with my inner Self that I had achieved this evening was the most important thing in life. The investment I have long carried to "save the world" was an escape from doing what I needed to realize myself. The world doesn't need saving; anyone who wishes to be saved need only turn to the Source for full guidance. Everything is in the best of all possible hands. Becoming united with the deep Self is by far the most important and wonderful thing anyone can do. I reveled in my feeling of love for Jean, and knew that our life will be better than ever.

I was unable to sleep at all that night, but worked the entire time. What I was experiencing was so rejuvenating that I felt rested. By morning I felt an enormous wholeness and peace within me. It was as though the struggle of a whole lifetime had come to a marvelous, fabulous fruition. I was astounded at the quantum leap in understanding, at the amazing amount of wisdom that came to me, and the enormous speed at which it came. I felt that at last I was beginning to use these substances properly. Employing trust and surrendering to the Inner Teacher, there is no end to the learning that can be accomplished.

When I arose in the morning, I had never felt so whole, so centered, and so confident in my entire life. I was egoless, ready to deal with each moment, whatever it demanded.

That day we drove to Death Valley and back with two close friends. I drove the entire distance. Our trip was a continuation of my experience. Using the same approach of surrendering to Trust, I continued my experience and the surrounding beauty rose to incredible heights. At the peak of the experience I found that I could think in an entirely new way. I entered a state that I would call gnosis, where everything that I looked at seemed utter truth, directly from the Source.

As I explored realization at this level, the feeling of union with gnosis became more and more powerful, until I was literally merged in the wonder of the central light. It confirmed all of life, and gave complete assurance that absolutely everything is being taken care of perfectly. At this level, everything is perfect – absolutely clean and pure. No dross can be carried into this area. In this light, one is perfectly cleansed. I need only be open for instructions of what is best to do and the knowledge will be forthcoming.

Everyone is part of this wonderful whole, pursuing their own course in life as they wish. Each person can partake of the whole to the extent that he or she wishes. Again, I need not be concerned about the progress of others, other than to be helpful when requested, as each is free to explore his or her own diversity of experience. They move according to their own choice.

Despite having had no sleep the night before, I arrived home full of energy. Others were ready to relieve me, but anytime I felt tired, I simply released to experience and became revitalized.

I was overwhelmed by the impact of this experience. It takes an enormous stretching of the mind to fully appreciate the wonders and grace I had received. I had been freed of much of the unnecessary baggage I had been carrying, I had been shown how to become free, I had been privileged to enter that extraordinary Clear Light that must be the ultimate experience for man. But most of all, I had been thoroughly shown the utter reality of the Source that underlies creation, and that the most important thing one can do with one's life is place one's implicit trust in this Source. Certainly I had the key to successfully living the remainder of my life.

So it was with great disappointment that I discovered in the weeks that followed that this experience faded into memory like those before. The outstanding feeling of well-being, the ability to rapidly clear whatever might be bothering me, faded away. Many of my old habits returned, including the ability to sink into tiredness and depression. The depression was accentuated by the realization that finding such a significant answer was not the total answer.

Yet something was different. As the weeks rolled by, I found that I had discovered something priceless. There was something to trust, and I began to learn how to surrender to it from the ordinary state of consciousness. The knowledge I had found had deeply penetrated my being. It was available to be used. I needed to learn how to train my ordinary being to recognize and utilize the wisdom. I found myself dealing more effectively with my problems and bringing about changes in my life. The knowledge was seeping through into my life, but required my conscious cooperation!

The ultimate result of this outstanding experience was a significant leap forward in all of my subsequent exploration with the sacraments, as well as in my meditation practice. All of my experiences became more meaningful, with a steady progression of each being better than the last. I was learning to move into new territory, find greater joy and wisdom in the experiences, and more effectively make changes.

Research with new compounds continued until the passage of the Controlled Substance Analogue Enforcement Act of 1986, which effectively makes every psychoactive drug illegal before it is even invented.[1]

Fear of the unconscious is so deeply set in our current society that we have now made every substance illegal which has any promise of revealing unconscious material. Such fear includes resisting knowledge of the depth and power of the human mind, as well as spiritual realities.

One cannot help but ponder the strange dichotomy that the nation based on establishing individual freedom has now outlawed every substance which might aid in the exploration of that last and most important frontier, the human mind. Alexander Shulgin, world-renowned chemist in the field of psychoactive drugs, is quoted in a recent periodical: "Our generation is the first ever to have made the search for self-awareness a crime."[2]

The most penetrating, insightful, informed, and thoroughly researched discussion of our current drug laws of which I am aware is presented by Jonathan Ott in the introductory chapter to his book *Pharmacotheon*[3] entitled Proemium. Our irrational and destructive drug laws are scholarly reviewed from the perspectives of science, practical and legal considerations, morality, economics, and coping with ecstasy and euphoria.

The widespread fear of the unconscious contents of our minds will be overcome as people learn the value of confronting and regaining the power and wisdom locked up in repressed feelings and dynamics. With the removal of the barriers of repressed material, the enormous range of innate human capacities can be discovered and developed. Characteristics such as intuition, creativity, freedom of thought, and heightened perception can be developed. Inspiration, peace, and the capacity to love can be drawn from the discovery of the transcendental levels of consciousness.

Psychedelics are a powerful tool which, when skillfully applied by motivated seekers, can significantly help accomplish all of the above. Much of the research work that I and other investigators have done with psychedelic compounds over the last three decades confirms the potential of achieving the above results.

I shall devote the remainder of this volume to reporting some of the interesting information that has been revealed in our studies.

Most of the reports of experiences in this book are my own. Consequently they are a reflection of my own dynamics. Compared to other explorers whom I know, I have spent much more time exploring negative feelings. I am not sure of all the reasons – whether it's unresolved, deep layers of conditioning, an unusual sensitivity whereby I am innately aware of other people's pain, the perfectionism of my aspirations, or my pig-headed stubbornness to change. The fact remains that I have learned much about dealing with shadow material. In the end, despite the discomfort, this has been extremely rewarding, and well worth any pain involved. I have followed the Buddhist principle of dealing with adversity and turning it into opportunity for spiritual growth.

The biggest problem I encountered was my inability to maintain the exalted states I was privileged to experience. This became most evident as I reviewed the records for this writing. Putting these experiences in perspective by writing about them has helped a great deal in recognizing the need and deepening the intention to make changes. Some additional explanation may be helpful in perusing the reports presented.

I refer frequently throughout my reports to feelings which I call "crud", "psychic junk", or "loading". The term "negative karma" is the Eastern designation for such feelings. See Chapter 3, Note 4, for an explanation of karma.

Such feelings are depressing, uncomfortable, even painful. They feel to me like a heavy weight the body is carrying. They build what feels like a tangible wall between me and the world around me. This wall sometimes gets thick enough to limit the details I can see and feel of my surroundings. These miserable feelings demand attention and often draw me into introspection to seek resolution. Such withdrawal further separates me from others and my surroundings.

There are two major sources, I believe, for the continued build-up of these uncomfortable feelings. The first is the consequence of everyday activities, and results primarily from not behaving authentically. In my case, where it has meant a great deal to have approval, I have repressed behavior which I think may not be accepted (repressing is an unconscious process, to be distinguished from consciously deciding to behave in a certain manner). It is most often anger and resentment that I repress, not wishing to show it. This results in further repressed anger, as there is a part of me that hates myself for not being honest. This adds to the load. There are other things that I repress in order to not affect the image I wish to present to others.

A factor which very much determines how much we repress is our aspirations. In my case, I wish to become as free as possible, and to continue my growth until I achieve complete liberation (see Appendix IV for a definition of this state). As awareness grows, there is heightened joy and heightened appreciation of all aspects of life. But the greater awareness also permits us to observe with greater clarity our own difficulties and those of others.

This heightened awareness can be a source of dissatisfaction. So it behooves us to be quite clear on how far and how fast we wish to develop. Greater clarity means taking on more responsibility, and we must be certain that this is what we wish to do. Change is difficult, and once we know that we should, avoiding it is painful. This is another reason that the use of psychedelic substances should be carefully evaluated, and why they should be taken with clear intention.

Many areas were difficult for me to change, particularly in my marriage relationship. Each experience has been a clear reminder of the necessity to take responsibility and work at producing the required changes if I wish to retain the exalted states.

The unresolved difficulties in my marriage have been a key element in the return of miserable feelings. These are dealt with specifically in Chapter 14, The Story of a Marriage.

The second cause of uncomfortable feelings is the surfacing of feelings that have been repressed from early life experience. I see these as layers and layers of unconscious conditioning, which go deeply to the very core of the Self. In my experience, the deeper we go, the more solid the layers. The very bottom or most fundamental layers are extremely solid and heavily defended. These comprise the basic structure of our personality.

I doubt if many people attempt to reach and understand these layers, accepting them as the given part of themselves. Only if one aspires to true liberation as experienced and espoused by the Buddha, or from the Western viewpoint, mystical union with God (again, see Appendix IV for further clarification), will these layers be confronted and resolved. In my own case, I was aware of penetrating more deeply into the root core of my conditioning with ongoing experiences.

I ultimately found a deep, bitter, hostile part of myself. It was determined to thwart every gain in enjoyment. This bitter part of me is the source of thanatos, the drive for death. I ultimately had to make this hostile core my friend, and elicit its aid to achieve eros, the drive for life.

It is questionable if mainstream society understands or appreciates the extent of these layers of conditioning. I have given a description of them in Appendix IV, The Nature of the Self. I hope this Appendix will also help in understanding some of the experiences that are described in subsequent chapters.

To further appreciate the depth and toughness of these layers of conditioning, the following metaphor may permit a glimpse of the extent and power of them:

Assume the following characteristics of a completely liberated being: He/she perceives the surrounding world lit up with incredible light and beauty. Everything is charged with significance, and alive with energy. There is no awareness of any boundary to the self; the sense of self extends to encompass all that one can envision. The feeling tone is utter bliss, peace, and the most fulfilling contentment. This is the state of the natural self.

Now check your own feelings and perceptions. The difference between what you perceive and feel and the above description is the result of your true, inner self being surrounded by layers of conditioning. It is only by dissolving these layers that you can begin to experience the states described above for a liberated being.

Another example: In my experience, God is utterly real. When I am able to look Him in the face, the experience is as described by Meister Ekhart (see Appendix IV, Note 2). The light is so brilliant and the beauty so overwhelming that it is almost impossible to behold. Yet many are convinced that God does not exist at all, as they experience not a whit of evidence for His presence. It is testimony to the power of our minds that this overwhelming energy, light, and beauty can be completely nullified to the extent that we claim it does not exist. Yet this same power can be reversed, permitting us to perceive that we live in the Garden of Eden.

The information that follows in succeeding chapters has been selected to illustrate the enormous range and variety of experiences available from an informed use of psychedelic substances. Procedures for conducting explorations are described in Appendix III.

### Chapter 2 Notes

1. The Controlled Substance Analogue Enforcement Act of 1986 declares that any drug intended for human consumption

   which is substantially similar in chemical structure to –

or has stimulant, depressant, or hallucinogenic effects on the central nervous system that are substantially similar to or greater than –

or is represented or intended by a person to have stimulant, depressant, or hallucinogenic effects that are substantially similar to or greater than –

a substance in Schedule I or Schedule II shall be in Schedule I.

Because of the large number and variety of substances in Schedule I and Schedule II, it is extremely difficult to create a new psychoactive drug that is not "substantially similar" to a drug in these schedules. Thus the practical effect of this bill is to make it illegal to possess *any* psychedelic drug, now or in the future.

2. *Common Boundary*. January/February 1993, p. 32.
3. Ott, Jonathan. *Pharmacotheon*. Kennewick, WA: Natural Products Co., 1993, pp. 19-77.

# Chapter 3
# MDMA

For those who have been privileged to enter the sacred regions and appreciate the vast array of learning at our disposal, the psychedelics are priceless substances. But one stands out as especially unique, with outstanding characteristics exclusively its own. This is MDMA, code name for 3,4-methylenedioxy-N-methylamphetamine.[1] The most fitting description that I can give it is that it is an outstanding Grace.

David Nichols[2] has suggested a new class for this and similar acting substances, recommending the name entactogens – substances which allow "touching within". Ralph Metzner, in a paper "Psychedelics and Spirituality" delivered at a 1983 conference in Santa Barbara, has suggested the name empathogens – substances which bring one closer to oneself and others.

MDMA is not hallucinogenic like other psychedelics. It is in most cases quite euphoric, bringing about a sense of peace, wholeness, and well-being to the participant. It permits one to see the world in an exciting new way, alive with energy, color, and euphoria. And remarkably, these responses are quite uniform over a wide range of participants.

This characteristic of uniformity is quite different from other psychedelics, where an enormous range of responses is possible. Results with the most active psychedelics depend on a variety of factors such as the subject's individual value system, the state of his/her psyche, the subject's aspirations, and the setting for the experience, including the character of the companions present. While these factors are also important for MDMA, the action of the drug considerably overrides their influence, providing a much wider range of acceptance for suitable candidates.

I will never forget my own introduction to MDMA. I was still in the stage where every psychedelic experience started with several hours of discomfort, as I previously reported in Chapter 2. This was the first time this did not happen to me. Once the drug took effect, there was a marvelous energy rush, and I was in a state of euphoria! Everything around me was delightfully infused with light and energy. Never had I so enjoyed an experience. Observing that I was well into the effects, my sponsor came over and said to me something that I shall never forget: "Welcome to my world!" And what a world it was. A beautiful, loving, euphoric world free of the dead serious learning and striving I had always carried with me into these journeys. A world alive with light, energy, meaning, and especially love.

MDMA was a great discovery, and Jean and I immediately began to study it more extensively. As we got more familiar with it, we began to define some of its characteristics.

While MDMA did not lend itself to introspection as readily as some other substances, it did permit a great deal of clarity and self-understanding if one were motivated to turn his/her attention in this direction. Problems were accurately perceived and their solutions apparent. There was a remarkable tendency when in this state to feel exceptionally whole and with no need to defend oneself. Participants could readily discuss differences with others with remarkable freedom and insight.

In a study that Charles Wells and I did on 2C-T-2 and 2C-T-7,1 we compared the first time use of those substances to the initial use of MDMA. We had this to say about MDMA in our paper:[3]

> MDMA has been widely used and reported upon. The most complete treatments are Adamson (1985)[4], Eisner (1989)[5], and Beck et al. (1989)[6]. Eisner (1989) contains a complete, annotated bibliography of the scientific literature on MDMA through 1988 (including a sampling of the popular literature) prepared by Dr. Alexander T. Shulgin. In our trials, we most often administered an initial dose of 120 m.g. followed by a 40 m.g. supplement at the one and one-half hour point to sustain the experience. This dose level seemed optimum with a surprisingly wide variety of subjects. We found the major characteristics to be a satisfying feeling of being centered and whole, a feeling of euphoria, freedom from uncomfortable or untoward responses once the full effect of the drug was established, a sense of inner security with no need to defend oneself, and an ability to look at oneself honestly and with detachment.

Our subjective observations of MDMA are reported in more detail in Chapter 14, Story of a Marriage.

After a number of trials of MDMA with other people, it became apparent that this was the best substance with which to introduce people to psychoactive drugs. With other substances, we had always used great care to make sure that the subject was ready for an experience that would greatly alter his perceptions, understanding, and perhaps his view of himself and his behavior. MDMA is so generally euphoric and non-threatening that a much wider range of subjects can benefit from the experience without discomfort.

We were privileged to have so useful a tool, and extended our study of it to a number of people. One area of application that was particularly satisfying was with our family. We were extremely gratified with the level of bonding that resulted from sharing MDMA with different family members. Even my older brother, who was a particular nemesis of mine in my childhood, consented to share the experience. While he never became an advocate, he enjoyed the experience. Joining him permitted me to drop some ancient grievances for the bullying I had received as a younger brother, and allowed me to perceive him in a warm, new light. While advancing years alone can produce maturity that enhances closeness, this experience created a bond that shall always remain.

While sharing the experience of MDMA with close family and friends was always satisfying, we began to become aware of a limitation. The experience was most enjoyable and very centering. Yet it did not open the doors to a wide range of exploration as effectively as other psychedelic substances.

Another disadvantage was the large amount of chemical ingested. This produced some toxic side-reactions, such as jaw-clenching and muscle tensions. We found that continued use of MDMA gradually eliminated these side-effects, as though the causes were being dissolved away through additional experiences.[7] Even so, the aftermath was not the same as with the established psychedelics such as LSD and mescaline, which most often leave the body quite cleansed and rejuvenated.

MDMA is short acting, reaching a peak in one hour, and beginning to decline in another thirty minutes. A supplement at this 1-1/2 hour point of approximately 1/3 of the original dose will keep the experience going at peak intensity for another hour or so (others have reported that a two hour wait to supplement is more satisfactory). But once the effect wears off, the activity suddenly drops.

If one's psyche is relatively clear, the descent is quite euphoric, and the remainder of the day is spent in a very satisfying state of contentment.

However, if there is unresolved material in the unconscious that did not get dealt with completely, the drop in the action of the drug seems quite sudden, and one is left physically uncomfortable and somewhat unsettled.

To counteract this we thought, why not supplement with another, more powerful substance? This turned out to be a splendid idea. I particularly liked it, because what made the beginning of my psychedelic explorations uncomfortable was the negative karma[8] I had accumulated, which had to be expiated before I could thoroughly enjoy the experience. Now I could dispose of this with MDMA, which occurred, I felt, automatically and very pleasantly. So when I took the additional substance, I was ready to soar into fresh spaces free of my usual psychic load.

This worked very effectively. In fact, everyone invariably reported that their experience with the psychedelic supplement was better than using that particular substance alone. MDMA is an empowering launching pad.

This worked so well that I embarked on a study to prove that *every* good psychedelic was better if first preceded by MDMA. It didn't matter whether the psychedelic was ingested at the normal supplement time, one hour and thirty minutes after ingesting the MDMA, or an hour or so after taking the normal supplement of MDMA. People often preferred the latter just to enjoy the MDMA state longer, and then go into the somewhat different experience provided by the second drug.

Unfortunately, this investigation was never carried to a conclusion because of the temporary placing of MDMA in Schedule I of the Controlled Substances Act in 1985. MDMA was permanently made a Schedule I substance in 1988. It did give us time to find out that LSD, 2-CB, MEM, and 2C-T-2 were all enhanced when MDMA was taken first. We felt that MDMA and MEM was a particularly powerful combination for one earnestly seeking solution of his/her problems. More data on this last combination is reported in Chapter 5.

The procedure of starting first with MDMA might not have as much benefit for experienced explorers.

Because of the efficacy of combining MDMA with other substances, we focused our attention on these combinations for a period of time. Except for one report covering the combination of MDMA and LSD, this work is reported in the chapters covering the second drug.

At times when administering MDMA, Jean and/or I would choose a different substance to accompany the participants. In my own case, I was suffering from prostatitis. The extreme dehydration resulting from the ingestion of MDMA made urinating difficult even with copious amounts of water. It also caused painful urinary irritation. As this malady grew worse, painful urination would last as long as a week after an MDMA experience. And with frequent experiences, it was well to avoid the discomfort of the greater toxic after-effects of MDMA.

We found that a dose of 16 m.g. of 2C-B would allow us to enter the same space as those on MDMA and participate fully in their experience. It was unnecessary to take a supplement, and the descent and after effects were much improved. Still later, we found 2C-T-2 even more satisfactory, and it would remain active for a longer period of time. Doses of 8 m.g. to 12 m.g. are effective, depending on the psychic burden of the group (those weighted down with problems absorb more energy).

Undergoing a transurethral resection of the prostate completely eliminated the urinary problem with MDMA. However, by this time I had learned to use 2C-B or 2C-T-2 to obtain all the benefits of MDMA. These two drugs also permitted greater freedom in exploring other levels of thought and feeling. So I abandoned MDMA except for special occasions.

The scheduling of MDMA took place in 1985. Although set aside by an appeal, it became permanently scheduled in 1988, and remains so to this time. The legal ramifications leading to the scheduling of MDMA are covered by Bruce Eisner,[5] pages 26 to 31. The references in the notes of this chapter describe a wide array of experiences with MDMA. Below are a few excerpts from our own experience. For the most part, these experiences were conducted unstructured, simply observing how different persons would react. Carefully preparing the subjects, focusing the experience through serious intention on the part of the participants, and repeating the experience to further the results would considerably enhance the outcome.

### *A Sudden Shift*

This report indicates how rapidly strong negative feelings can be dissipated. Jean and I had tried MDMA only a few times when we moved to the high desert. Our enthusiasm for this new substance was so great that we were eager to share it with close friends.

Two weeks after our move, several friends were visiting us. Jean was not at all well, being worn out from our move and trying to fit our multitude of belongings into a smaller house. Her anxieties were compounded by having to play hostess before our house was properly settled. She reported that she was anxious, very depressed, and exhausted.

One astute visitor assessed her state, and suggested that we share MDMA. All agreed.

> Jean took 100 m.g., the rest of us 120 m.g. It was a beautiful fall day, and we all opened delightfully to the experience. Everyone's face became soft, young-looking, and took on a transcendental look. Jean became deeply relaxed, and

> all of her troubles melted away. The supplement deepened the experience and increased the bonding among us. We felt blessed to be together.
>
> The afterglow on the following day was outstanding. We had all been quite moved by the experience, and were reluctant to part. Jean had totally dropped the uncomfortable feelings of the previous morning. For the next few days she cheerfully undertook the considerable task of getting our home in order.

### *Recovering Her Voice*

We are visiting a young friend, Adele, who is an excellent singer, accompanying herself on the guitar. She has been quite run down, dropping in and out of the flu, and is very low in energy. This has resulted in a very raspy throat and she is unable to sing. She hopes an experience with MDMA will be helpful.

> Jean takes 100 m.g. of MDMA, Adele and I take 120 m.g. As the effect of the MDMA comes on, paintings on the wall come to life. The wallpaper is a dark gold; I see it getting very bright and attractive. I doubt if I shall ever see it dull again. I am intensely intoxicated, probably the deepest so far. Everyone's skin has softened; the two girls look radiant and beautiful. We all feel glorious.
>
> At the height of the experience, Adele decides to sing to us. She plays and sings perfectly. Her voice is angelic; there is no trace of the raspiness in her singing, or in her speaking voice. She discovers that she has been pushing herself too hard, and needs to take more time to relax.

### *Introspection*

Jean and I were introduced to MDMA in a group, and found group participation most rewarding. We loved the interchange, the freedom of communication, the bonding with others, often heightened by focusing the discussion on significant issues in our lives.

This was a welcome contrast to the directed, interior journey we employed in the Foundation days, and used by many other therapists. While the interior journey is most valuable in getting acquainted with yourself in all of its aspects, group interchange has much to offer in developing social skills and an appreciation of others.

I often became aware that I was not really listening to others. I learned a lot about how to truly listen, and how satisfying it is when others listen carefully to me. I also became aware of my discomforts and how to be at ease with others, especially those who knew a good deal more than I did.

This group participation was so very rewarding that it was difficult to consider using MDMA any other way. But one time when Jean and I were sharing an experience, she felt introspective. I used the silence to look around at the clouds and the mountains. I found that the quiet leads to a far different kind of experience, much more like LSD. I saw much imagery and great beauty in the clouds. I experienced profound realizations of the power of love and how it flows from the Source as the greatest of all gifts. And how our lives can be transformed in expressing it.

On a different occasion, in taking a walk around the property under the influence of MDMA (something we usually don't feel like doing), the surroundings lighted up with signifcance and meaning, just as with the more powerful psychedelics. It became clear that even though each substance has its own particular characteristics and tends to focus in particular areas, once one became proficient at utilizing that substance, it can with volition be directed in other useful ways.

### *A Young Couple*

Estelle is a classmate of my daughter at Occidental college. She and a friend of hers, Graham, are visiting us in the high desert. Both are quite spiritually oriented and practice meditation. They had both used LSD in their earlier days with mixed results, and had abandoned it. While they had discovered some of the higher levels of awareness they were seeking, they often got into uncomfortable spaces that made the experiences unrewarding. Now they are intrigued by our description of the new substance, MDMA, and wish to experience it.

> Estelle and Graham each take 100 m.g. of MDMA, Jean and I 120 m.g. Graham feels a powerful surge of energy and is riding a wave. The tension he usually feels with LSD is absent. He begins to glow brightly; there is nothing negative or painful. He reports a suspension of judgment and being more in the moment.
>
> Estelle experiences some resistance. She finally breaks through, and is all smiles. She had been afraid that I would try to control her experience, since I had been so ardent about the virtues of MDMA. She is quite relieved to find that I let her have her own experience, and thanks me. Graham reports that I had been a bit too strong for him also. Now we all feel quite intoxicated, enjoying the beauty, the joy of being with each other, the superb feeling of love, and the ease of sharing with each other.
>
> Estelle and Graham go for a long walk, thoroughly enjoying being outdoors, experiencing nature and deepening their relationship.
>
> Reviewing the experience, Estelle had not experienced much enhancement in vision or colors, but felt things more deeply. She particularly liked the outdoors, feeling the wind and experiencing smells. She felt that she worked through some barriers and very much enjoyed spending a day away from the intellect.
>
> Graham felt very open and that it was much safer to share. He felt very energetic and ready to frolic. He now has a greater appreciation of things and more primitive sensations.

As a result of this experience together, Estelle and Graham discovered how much they cared for each other, and some months later they were married. They now have two children and are pursuing successful careers.

We didn't hear much from them, although we were present at their wedding. About a year after, Graham confided in me. He apologized for not having expressed appreciation for the day we spent together. He wanted me to know that it was a turning point in their life and brought them together. For this they were both extremely grateful.

### *Face to Face With God*

Veronica is a beautiful young girl of 30 years, a close friend of my son and his wife. She is a very sensitive person, and has a talent for channeling other levels of awareness. In the past she has been intimidated at the prospect of using psychedelics, but at last felt she was ready for an experience. Because of her sensitiveness, she starts with a lighter dose of 100 m.g. of MDMA:

> She had a remarkable breakthrough. She was positive that she was going to die, so she decided to let herself die. She melted into the ground, and then appeared before a profound, brilliant light, the throne of God. She knew that she was with God, and that she *was* God. She was in ecstasy, and began to sing. She turned into a delightful little girl, utterly alive, bright, full of joy and wisdom. She was so beautiful, inside and out, that she was a joy to witness. She felt her channel was wide open directly to the Source and was extremely insightful about whatever subject took our attention.
>
> We all take a 40 m.g. supplement of MDMA, and the experience continues in the same vein for the next two hours. We all feel remarkably rejuvenated, and exult in the marvel of this experience.

About a year later we see Veronica again. She has had a miscarriage at three months.

She not only is suffering the loss of her child, but underwent some painful medical procedures. She is visiting to recuperate and would like another MDMA experience.

> Veronica takes 100 m.g. of MDMA. Jean and I monitor on 16 m.g. each of 2C-B. As Veronica gets into the experience, she cries over the pain of her loss. She has always feared the death of someone close. But now things are changing. She sees the loss as a gift. Life and death are the same – the problems are our attachments, what we think we want. God is present in the deepest pain. There is nothing but love. Life is so beautiful, so vast. We are never given more than we can handle. Life is never cruel; we are forced to open up to look. God loves us so much.
>
> Veronica continues, life means so much more when we experience death, especially the death of the ego. Veronica feels one with all women. Heavy karma is now a blessing. Everything is more alive. It is a blessing to be a woman. This has been a most rewarding experience.

### *Freeing the Body*

Veronica has made excellent use of her MDMA experiences, but does not choose to use psychedelics frequently. Her next experience is seven months later. Visiting us in our son's home, she suddenly realizes how much she yearns for another experience, as she is carrying an overwhelming load.

Veronica takes 110 m.g. of MDMA. As she gets into it, she requests my assistance with Focusing. This is a procedure developed by Eugene T. Gendlin; it is fully described in his book entitled *Focusing*.[9] I have found this to be one of the most effective means I know to contact and release hidden feelings, and particularly to relieve the body of stress.

I lead her in the process, encouraging her to alternately feel without resisting the feeling she has chosen to examine and then find the most appropriate handle – a word, phrase, or image that best describes the feeling – as described in Gendlin's book. The action of the MDMA accelerates this process, and she responds dramatically. Her body expresses itself. It feels tired, neglected, unlistened to, pushed around. Veronica has not listened to her body for years. She loves her body, but there is much control, which produces stress. There are many people who depend on her; although she loves to nurture others, she has been overdoing it and has been neglecting her body. Now it is unhappy and alone. She finds that she doesn't forgive easily, but holds things close to her chest. She particularly wants noted in the record, FORGIVENESS IS THE ANSWER TO SADNESS. Now her body feels great because she has been listening to it.

## *A Very Special Day*

Sophia has been a good friend since the days of the Foundation. She went through our program, and it made a very significant impact on her life. She redirected her life into spiritual growth. In the intervening years, she has made outstanding progress and has been a great source of inspiration for many whom she teaches. Her husband Gregory also has deep spiritual interests and is an excellent scholar.

Sophia had lately been pondering the advantage of another trial of the sacraments. She was delighted to hear of the new substance, MDMA, and Jean and I agreed to travel to their home to join them in an exploration.

I arrived the sickest I had been in over a year. I had a miserable case of the flu – dizziness, aching bones, extreme tiredness, deep chest cough, and congestion. I wondered how I could proceed with an experience. Yet we had traveled a great distance, and felt that introducing Sophia and Gregory to MDMA was such a promising opportunity that I could not refuse.

It was gratifying to see Sophia again and meet Gregory. We spent an evening visiting, and set the following day for our journey.

We start by taking 120 m.g. each of MDMA on an empty stomach. In twenty-seven minutes my head is clearing up miraculously. The congestion is disappearing, my sinuses open and I breathe clearly. After another twenty minutes, all the other bodily symptoms of my illness disappear and don't return all day!

The experience comes on strongly. We have learned that this intensity occurs with exceptionally good companions. We all move into an outstanding, euphoric state. We are enormously gratified to be with each other. We feel light, our voices are melodic, the skin smoothes and drops away the years, there is an outstanding feeling of grace. We quietly enjoy easy communication. It is snowing outside, and we feel very cozy together. I feel a deep sense of Presence.

Sophia reports that the simplest blade of grass is as important as the huge, distant mountain. Everything is all the same.

Gregory feels some self-doubt. He hadn't realized how invested he had become in a serious project he is undertaking and how it pushes him.

We all take a 40 m.g. supplement. We proceed blissfully. It goes so well that at the sign of wearing off, Sophia and Gregory ask for another supplement. I am leery, as past experience has shown the uncomfortable effects of the second supplement outweigh any benefits. But we feel so very good that we decide to do it anyway. The experience continues delightfully and we notice no ill effects. In fact, it is the richest, smoothest descent I have yet had from MDMA. Jean and I keenly feel the goodness of our host and hostess. [Because of the excellent result here, in a later investigation we once more tried a second supplement of MDMA. This second time it only proved our original premise, that the second supplement is not worthwhile except in very optimum circumstances.]

In the afternoon, Sophia reports that she has been spending the time making wider and wider circles, each time including more within the circle. Pain is the result of leaving something outside the circle. Gregory was aware of what she was doing. She faced all of her fears, including the death of her husband and her children. She knows that all is well. We are all elated with this experience.

The following day finds us all very mellow. Some of my flu symptoms return, but at a much lower level. It is mostly just tiredness. Gregory has encountered some vexing problems in his work situation, and finds that he handles them with considerably more balance and detachment.

As Sophia drove us to the airport the second day after our journey, I found myself moving into a new state of celestial grace I had never before experienced. In English we do not have an adequate vocabulary to deal with higher states of awareness, nor the experience to identify them. I can only report that this level seemed somehow more pristine, more sacred, so much further beyond my usual ways of perceiving and feeling as to represent an entirely different level of celestial existence. I was speechless; I could only hold still and be absorbed in this magnificent occurrence. I somehow knew that this enraptured state I had entered was related to the exceptional goodness of Sophia.

## *Pathology*

Jean and I were continually seeking suitable research subjects to extend our knowledge of the chemicals we were researching. Mostly we were looking for interested, stable individuals whom we thought could well handle and enjoy the experience. So I had to consider carefully when we were contacted by a college teacher who had been referred by a knowledgeable friend.

The biographical data I had requested revealed a scattered, disorganized person with serious family problems. This data, and the fact that his spouse did not wish to accompany him, were strong grounds for rejection. But he was very persistent. I was intrigued by our friend's assessment that we could be of help, even though years of conventional therapy had failed. I also wanted to extend our experience into this area. So we accepted.

Rudolpho, Jean and I each take 120 m.g. of MDMA. The experience develops slowly, like a balloon lifting a heavy weight. As the experience develops, Rudolpho shows us a photo album. It contains not only pictures of his family, but a number of girl friends he has slept with. In a short time he is extremely nauseous, and barely makes it to the john in time to vomit. His face is quite gray. He reports that he feels relieved from vomiting.

I ask him what the vomiting is about. He doesn't like his behavior, and doesn't want the double standard in his marriage. He feels he knows what it is like to be his son, from whom he is estranged and who has some serious emotional problems.

Rudolpho now feels quite relieved, and enjoys sitting in the sun. At supplement time, I suggest a larger supplement for him, as I feel he has much to deal with. He declines, and reluctantly accepts the normal 40 m.g. supplement. He is now feeling so good that he sees no need to take a supplement. He agrees only after I tell him the effects will soon wear off without a supplement, and that the supplement will simply continue the state he is in now, not intensify it.

Rudolfo refuses to look at his central problem, but delights in being the center of attention and running on and on verbally. In many years of Freudian psychoanalysis, he has learned to free associate. He does this for the next few hours, rambling freely over feelings, thoughts, and perceptions, totally uninterested in our responses or remarks. We listen for an hour, then remind him that the active part of the session will soon be over, and ask if he would like to address his problems. He can hold his attention on them for only a few seconds before he wanders away. After several unsuccessful attempts to redirect his focus, I realize that he is not going to attend his real issues, and we resign ourselves to listening. I am awed at the depth of his self-centeredness. Otherwise, we are all feeling quite good.

I am very surprised later in the day when the heavy burden I feel Rudolfo is carrying lifts and is replaced by a very satisfying euphoria. At this point Rudolfo feels normal and extremely clear-headed. He asks my evaluation of his experience. Earlier I had not wished to interfere with the spontaneous unfolding of his experience. Now I begin to share my perceptions of how he has utilized the experience. He seems open and understanding, so I feel he may wish to consider what I see are two of his major problems. However, he has little ability to stay focused on an issue. I spend the rest of the time reflecting back his behavior in the moment so he can learn to catch himself at what he is doing to disrupt relationships. Jean and I share our feelings and perceptions. These center on his inability to listen, his total selfabsorption to the point of ignoring others and opportunities to learn, and the importance of acknowledging and appreciating others. We hope some of it will seep through. The discussion continues through the next day.

We have no data as to the overall impact of this experience, and whether Rudolfo was able to improve the dynamics of his family relationships. He left us much happier, content, and with apparently more understanding. Jean and I learned a great deal about how distorted mental states can become, the power of investment in arbitrary belief systems, and how difficult it is to make inroads into them. Working with Rudolpho considerably improved the relationship between Jean and me. Seeing how bad things can get, she could acknowledge how much I had improved in overcoming some of the symptoms Rudolfo exhibited!

## *Focusing Energy*

Ted is a bright young man, 31 years old. On meeting, we soon found that we shared a great interest in psychedelics. Ted had used them frequently and quite constructively. As a result of what he learned in experiences, he decided on a career in the field of healing. He first went back to finish college, and is now working on an advanced degree which will aid him toward his goal. He plans to learn as much as possible through conventional study, and then use psychedelics to expand the frontiers of his knowledge. I admire the course he has chosen, as I feel that this is the ideal way for young people who experiment with psychedelics to utilize these substances.

We felt MDMA would be an appropriate substance to further our relationship.

> We all take 120 m.g. of MDMA. Ted responds very quickly; Jean and I follow somewhat later. It is an excellent takeoff. The experience grows beautifully, as Ted is an excellent person to be with.
>
> We are developing a great deal of energy, more than I have previously experienced with MDMA. Drawing on his knowledge of Hatha Yoga, Ted advises us to sit up straight, which focuses the energy. Ted uses his yoga exercises to direct the energy into an uplifting experence. After we all take a 40 m.g. supplement, Ted shows us how to breathe in, stretch and become very open to let the energy in, then deplete the breath. Following this procedure we get very energized.
>
> Ted then advises us to find a place in the body that feels good, and focus on increasing the good feeling. I find this very effective in directing the experience positively. I discover a choice point between letting the experience follow old normal patterns which get me into heavy feelings versus directing attention outward into new, exciting possibilities. I find this process of letting the body express good feelings and then amplifying them a very effective way to dissipate the bogged down feelings I often encounter, and which I am experiencing a bit here. This procedure of expanding the good feeling produces an ecstatic state.
>
> Later I make the surprising discovery that as long as I am directing my attention and working on something, the bliss inside continues to grow. Previously I had always thought that it was flowing love that dissipated interior discomfort and created bliss; now it seems to be blissful regardless of what I focus on, as long as it is worthwhile.
>
> We are all surprised by how this focusing activity has prolonged the experience and kept us in an advantageous space. That evening I feel the strongest and most secure yet on MDMA. Ted has been an excellent teacher.

I am putting these reports together several years after this experience took place. I must confess that I have not remembered this technique well enough to apply it in later experiences.

In the main, I have opted to directly confront my feelings and resolve them. This leaves me free, energized, and more knowledgeable. As I review this experience, it is clear that the procedures recommended by Ted are worth further exploration.

Sarah and John are a couple that I had known many years previously. They returned into our life seeking a psychedelic experience. I felt that MDMA, which we were just beginning to research, would be appropriate for them.

John is a fascinating person. He is deeply steeped in Eastern religions. But he lives a great deal in imagination, and is quite impervious to input from others. Sarah is a dedicated wife as dictated by her European culture, but has long since given up trying to receive cooperation or support from John. Her anger has grown to the extent that she hardly listens to anything he says. She is usually quiet and withdrawn, suffering in silence.

> We all take 120 m.g. of MDMA. In 45 minutes, Sarah becomes animated and begins to talk a lot. She also begins listening carefully to John. It isn't always easy to listen to him, as his explanations are circuitous and drawn out; it requires a lot of patience. Sarah grows in strength and begins to express many of her concerns.
>
> After a 40 m.g. supplement, we are in a good space, talking freely and easily. We spend the entire day simply talking and relating. Sarah and John develop a new appreciation of each other. Sarah notices something she has never experienced before. She had always thought that John rambled on and on repetitiously without making any sense. Now as she listens carefully, she is fascinated by his speech. She notices an aliveness, a charm, and an insightfulness that had escaped her. Her concentration makes it easier for her to understand what he is getting at, and she develops a true appreciation for a lot of the things he is discussing.
>
> As the day goes on, it becomes quite clear that John's defenses are ironclad, and that he has no desire to change. I work hard to get him to be more appreciative of Sarah and more cooperative. I reach a touchy boundary. John has had a great deal of rejection in his life; if I push too hard it could alienate him and he will withdraw. Yet it is to John's advantage to appreciate Sarah and give her space, so he can get some support back from her. John does notice that Sarah is changing, and fetches a mirror so that she can see it. I encourage him as much as I dare to take responsibility for Sarah's well-being.
>
> An excellent bond forms among us all. They have never been in such a salutary space, and are deeply appreciative of Jean and me. We spend the next day talking and reviewing. John and Sarah become very close and develop a good understanding between them. They feel better than they have in a long time, and are very grateful.

This experience opened the door for them to continue work on their relationship with other helpers and to support each other. They have both grown considerably over the following few years.

## *Wilbur and Donna*

Wilbur and Donna are both psychologists in their forties. They are of remarkably different temperaments. Wilbur is an extremely soft-spoken, highly sensitive, thoughtful person who keeps very much to himself. However, he doesn't hesitate to speak very forthrightly whenever he is moved, and is totally undaunted by whatever another person might think, regardless or in spite of their recognized stature.

Donna, on the other hand, is a total love. She is extremely open, outgoing, and a deeply caring person. They make a marvelous couple. They are both extremely bright and their attributes form an exquisite balance. With a common client they can play good guy – bad guy, Wilbur providing almost scathingly accurate, penetrating observations of a person's difficulties, while Donna provides the caring, nurturing support to help the client adjust to such realities.

In their youth they experimented with substances, but have not used them for a number of years. They are intrigued by the descriptions of MDMA, which hold forth promise of a valuable experience without the discomfort of encountering painful, suppressed material which had spoiled previous experiences. They decide to give it a try.

> Jean takes 110 m.g. of MDMA, the rest of us take 120 m.g. each. We are well into the experience in forty minutes, experiencing much euphoria, enthusiasm, youthful appearance, soft skin, easy communication, and enhanced beauty of perception. Wilbur is called to an inner exploration. He recalls an experience just before their marriage when an internal artery ruptured. Nevertheless he was in a state of bliss. He now feels this same bliss for the first time since that event. Also, Wilbur is pleased that a severe pain he has been experiencing in his arm is subsiding. He continues to search inside while the rest of us converse and listen to music.
>
> After a 40 m.g. supplement, we continue with great enjoyment, all being grateful for this very special time together. Wilbur reports that it is easy to look at his difficult areas and resolve them. He says, "you can look into the heart of anything". Donna also finds that the experience is valuable for uncovering things. She very much likes the centeredness and ability to focus, which is quite different from her mind-racing earlier experiences.
>
> I am very much aware of Wilbur's exceptionally fine mind and his enormous sensitivity. I tell him that he has immense potential.
>
> Two weeks later they repeated the experience on their own. It deeply cemented their relationship and understanding and acceptance of each other. Wilbur is very pleased with his new level of understanding, and Donna has made a quantum leap increase in aliveness. While I have always appreciated her as an extremely nurturing person, I find an enhanced physical interest in her as a female.
>
> They both felt that they had learned so much that it was unnecessary to repeat the experience.

### *Rebonding a Marriage*

Denise and Blake are a couple we met when they visited Dr. Wolff.[10] We shared many common values, and they were interested in our research. They had recently run into a very difficult situation in their marriage relationship, when one of them temporarily explored an alternate relationship. Although they reconciled, the warmth between them seems permanently affected. Hearing about the effectiveness of MDMA in relationships, they asked for a session.

Jean takes 110 m.g. of MDMA, Denise, Blake and I take 120 m.g. each. The experience quickly grows in intensity, which is typical with good people. Blake soon gets into a very good space. Within 30 minutes he is looking out of the window and seeing the mountains in great clarity, beauty, and depth. He is surprised at the depth because he sees well in only one eye. Then everything melts into one, and he experiences enormous peace and harmony. It is the experience of transcendence and oneness which he has actively sought, yet never before experienced. He wishes to dwell in this, but feels he should give his attention to Denise.

Denise at first feels somewhat unsettled by the onrush of energy. Then she is amazed to find herself experiencing incredible love for Blake. They fall into each other's arms with overwhelming love and deep bonding.

The remainder of the day they find themselves as youngsters in fresh young love, and explore the various dimensions of courtship. They are enthralled with each other and deeply connected. After a while their friends come into consciousness and are invited into their circle of love. Later Blake experiences Jesus, Buddha, and other dignitaries joining them and supporting them.

This experience brought Denise and Blake together in closeness as they had never thought possible. Their past difficulties were dissolved, and they continued their relationship in their new bond of love. They were enormously grateful for this experience. It made such an impact they have never felt it necessary to have another.

### *MDMA Plus LSD*

The combination of MDMA followed by LSD proved an extremely effective one. Here is an outstanding experience, one of the subject's very best:

Ernesto is a young medical student doing intern work at a nearby hospital. He had proven himself to be a very able user of the sacraments, and we have invited him and his wife Reina to join us for this research trial on a combination which is showing promise.

We all take 120 m.g. of MDMA on an empty stomach. Our closeness has grown through several shared experiences, and now we are all more intoxicated than ever. We are glowing, experiencing good feelings, animation, melodic voices, and expressive, youthful countenances. We are very insightful as we discuss people that we know.

At an hour and thirty-four minutes later, we each take 50 micrograms of LSD. We begin to quiet down in 20 minutes and put on music. Jean and Reina continue in the same beautiful state they were experiencing with MDMA.

Ernesto and I both begin to slide as the LSD comes on. I feel the marvelous glow of centeredness and euphoria slipping away, a "thinning out". It doesn't last long with Ernesto. The thinning stops, and his body becomes more light and expanded. His vision is clear, more profound, and with greater detail.

This is the outstanding experience of Ernesto's life. At the height of his experience he finds within himself a glowing ball of sheer power and love radiating with a white light. This is the source of life. He sees the same glowing ball in others.

Ernesto and Reina go off by themselves. They return later, and Ernesto appears an entirely new person. They had come together to seal their union, and after all the difficulties they had recently been through, it mobilized energy and shot Ernesto into a new space. He is totally aware, amazingly insightful and enormously confident. He is experiencing outstanding joy.

We have a wonderful interchange of discussion. At one point we mention meeting a girl who had taken the Transcendental Meditation course on levitation, and claimed that her hopping around the room was levitation. Ernesto is very exasperated that people should deceive themselves with such ideas when they have enormous power to develop themselves, improve their relationships, and be creative.

He asks Jean for a cup of tea, and she immediately rises to get it. "See", Ernesto says, "I levitated Jean. There are lots of things we can levitate".

Ernesto is aware of the enormous power we have within us, and that all we have to do is apply it correctly. Inspired by his positive approach, I look out the window and watch the light over the mountains which is the trail of the setting sun. This light grows into an enormous power, and I too see the vastness of the central power of the universe, and how it flows out in love. All traces of negative feelings within me evaporate and the rest of the day is blissful.

I put on for Ernesto the selection from Handel's Messiah, A Son is Born. It strikes him with enormous impact, as well as the rest of us.

Ernesto had previously had strong misgivings about leaving Mexico and his family. He is now able to truly appreciate the United States and what it means to have a nation devoted to the freedom of the individual. The impact of our nation's values affects the whole world. I play a Fred Waring rendition of Give Me Your Tired, Your Poor. The real meaning of our nation, opening the golden gates to the underprivileged of the world and offering them fresh opportunity, strikes us dramatically. We are all overwhelmed with emotion. What a loss it is to lose sight of our high principles by getting involved in the piddly affairs of everyday life.

Ernesto had an interesting experience after returning to the hospital. He reported that work flowed beautifully and insightfully, and saw many ways in which the inner power can be expressed in life.

At one point, he got a feeling he should go to the Emergency Room. There a doctor and two nurses were trying to insert an IV into an elderly diabetic. The patient was so dehydrated that they could not find a vein, and had punctured her in a great many places without success. Ernesto suggested to one of the nurses that she insert the needle where two veins came together, so she could strike the fork. The nurse laughed, knowing Ernesto as a fresh, inexperienced intern, while she had inserted needles thousands of times. The doctor asked Ernesto to try. He inserted the needle successfully on the first try. The patient was enormously grateful. Ernesto felt that he had been called to the Emergency Room to help her.

Jean found this combination an outstanding experience. Under the impact of the LSD, she was entirely taken over by the music. She heard Dvorak's New World Symphony as though she had never heard it before. Each note danced inside and outside of her, and she became the notes.

At the height of the MDMA experience Reina felt herself as being all things. With the action of the LSD she began to bring everything back inside herself, finding a strong, inner core forming like a staunch rod. Her thoughts became profound, and she could see more clearly as she focused on her work and her relationships.

For me, I realized how very important it is to focus my thinking and attention, which directs my power. Then things flow readily and easily. I saw that a clear way out of my pain is to focus my energy into meaningful activities.

By usual standards, the amount of LSD which we imbibed was quite small. Yet the impact on all of us was extraordinary. For Ernesto, it was a rare +4 experience (see rating scale in Appendix II), a once-in-a-lifetime occurrence.

.......

These are only a few of the many rewarding experiences we had with MDMA. I wish to once more call attention to the fact that most of these experiences were unstructured.

Preparation, intentional focusing, and repeated trials can considerably improve results.

Recent information on MDMA is presented by Nicholas Saunders in his book *E for Ecstasy*.[11] Saunders has gathered all of the information he could find on MDMA. His book includes reviews of previously published material, as well as recent developments. Included in the latter are the rave scene in England, psychotherapeutic work in Switzerland, and research projects in Britain.

As for our own work, we believe that almost any one of the trials we conducted would convince an objective observer that MDMA is a substance which holds enormous promise for improving the quality of life, and richly deserves careful investigation. Becoming familiar with the full range of possibilities offered by this exceptional compound would make it hard to deny that it is one of life's remarkable graces.

### Chapter 3 Notes

1. The drugs 2C-T-2 and 2C-T-7 are code names for 2,5-dimethoxy-4- ethylthiophenethylamine and 2,5-dimethoxy-4-(n)-propylthiophenethylamine respectively. The synthetic procedures and physical characteristics of these compounds, as well as MDMA, are published in Shulgin, A. T. & Shulgin, A. *PIHKAL*. Berkeley, California: Transform Press, 1991.
2. Nichols, D. E. "Differences Between the Mechanisms of Action of MDMA, MBDB, and the Classic Hallucinogens. Identification of a New Therapeutic Class: Entactogens". *J. Psychoactive Drugs* 18:305-313, 1986.
3. Stolaroff, M. J. and Wells, C. W. "Preliminary Results with New Psychoactive Agents 2C-T-2 and 2C-T-7". Scheduled for publication in *Yearbook for Ethnomedicine and the Study of Consciousness*, Volume 2, 1994. Christian Rätsch, Editor.
4. Adamson, S. *Through the Gateway of the Heart*. San Francisco: Four Trees Publications, 1985.
5. Eisner, B. *Ecstasy: The MDMA Story*. Berkeley, CA.: Ronin Publishing, Inc., 1989.
6. Beck, J; Harlow, D.; McDonnell, D.; Morgan, P.A.; Rosenbaum, M.; & Watson, L. 1989. *Exploring Ecstasy: A Description of MDMA Users*. Institute for Scientific Analysis Final Report to the National Institute of Drug Abuse, 9/15/89.
7. My hypothesis, derived from thirty years of observation of some five hundred experiences, is that the ingestion of a psychedelic substance releases layers of material that have been repressed in the unconscious. The rate of release depends upon

the dose level, how heavily these layers are defended, the focus of attention, and the intent of the subject. But even with no focused attention, such layers are to some extent released, so that repeated experiences will continue the freeing process. The occluded areas in the unconscious demand attention and can be the source of uncomfortable feelings. Consequently as repeated experiences free these areas, the experience, and particularly the descent, becomes more comfortable, especially with MDMA.

8. Karma is a fundamental concept in Eastern thought, and is literally translated as action. It is held that our actions in life are influenced by our previous actions. Inappropriate actions in the past will result in current inappropriate actions or experiences, whereas good acts will result in further good acts and experiences. Jesus made a very similar statement, "As ye sow so shall ye reap".

   Extensive experience with psychedelics reveals the enormous amount of material we repress. It is this content that we attempt to resolve in dreams. Research has shown that preventing sleepers from dreaming by waking them when they show the rapid eye movements that are correlated to dreaming causes them to become irritable and disturbed. Some psychedelic experiences are like intense dreams as repressed material is released. Our first Foundation published paper, The Psychedelic Experience, A New Concept in Psychotherapy (see Appendix I for the reference), describes typical progress through successive stages of the experience. As the unconscious material is resolved, the meaning and significance of the imagery become more apparent. This correlates to dreams becoming more understandable and meaningful as we give them our conscious attention and work with them.

   I have chosen the term "negative karma" as an alternate way to describe inappropriate repressed material which must be resolved, or as Easterners would say, redeemed.

9. Eugene T. Gendlin. *Focusing*. New York: Bantam Books, 1981. Dr. Gendlin's book is a result of research at the University of Chicago to determine the factors that influence the rate of progress in therapy. This book incorporates procedures learned from that research, and I highly recommend it. The approach is intended to most rapidly and effectively elicit buried feelings and personal dynamics and resolve them. It combines willingness to feel the buried feelings with the use of the intellect to most rapidly zero in on the heart of the problem. The subject is advised how to allow feelings to come up without resistance. Then a "handle" is chosen – a word, phrase, or image that best describes the feeling. The subject then once again gives attention to the feeling. The handle is rechecked against the feeling to see if it is still the best fit. If not, it is changed. Attention is given alternately to focusing on the feeling and the most appropriate handle. In time a "felt shift" is experienced, which is the release of the feeling, often accompanied by valuable insights. Procedures are clearly and thoroughly explained in the book, with advice on how keep the process going and deal with obstacles or other developments.

10. Dr. Franklin Merrell-Wolff – philosopher, mathematician, mystic, and sage – is known for having achieved spontaneous states of enlightenment through five progressive 'Realizations.' He wrote of his experiences in great detail and clarity in his two books:

    *Pathways Through to Space: A Personal Record of Transformation in Consciousness*. New York: Richard Smith, 1942.

    *The Philosophy of Consciousness Without an Object: Reflections on the Nature of Transcendental Consciousness*. New York: Julian Press, 1973.

    Dr. Wolff lived the latter years of his life at the foot of the Sierra Nevada Mountains above Lone Pine, California. His three hundred acre estate included housing

where persons could come and stay and study his writings and extensive tape recordings and consult with him.
11. Saunders, Nicholas. *E for Ecstasy*. London: Nicholas Saunders, 1993.

# Chapter 4
# 2C-B

2C-B, code name for 4-bromo-2,5-dimethoxyphenethylamine[1], is one of the outstanding members of the phenethylamine family of psychoactive drugs. It is almost ten times as potent as MDMA, being active in the dose range of 12 to 30 m.g. It has its own unique characteristics, and for many is a great favorite. It is shorter acting than most of the full range psychedelics, lasting about six hours.

The characteristic for which it is most appreciated is the enhancing of the senses. It makes all of the senses more acute, greatly increasing the enjoyment of vision, touch, hearing, and taste. Many have been excited by the amplification of eroticism, and have found 2C-B a marvelous enhancer of love-making.

Jean and I usually found that we had so many resentments to work through that we did not fully appreciate 2C-B as a facilitator of lovemaking. However, when I have been able to enter what I consider the special 2C-B world, it is a delightful place. There is a subtlety of perception, a special way of appreciating nature. This enhanced sensitivity is very difficult to describe; perhaps the best word for it is tenderness. It is exquisite to experience and is unique to this substance. Sometimes it strikes me as if the highest qualities of a supreme feminine presence is everywhere manifest.

2C-B is not uniformly enjoyed. Only about half of those who have tried it report the favorable aspects I have described above. Many others found it made them quite uncomfortable in their bodies. I have known some that were so distressed that they don't care to try it again.

As we got familiar with it we experienced the body discomfort people complained about, but found we could work through that to the enjoyable aspects. On the suggestion of others that 2C-B makes you quite aware of your body, I formed the hypothesis that the uncomfortable feelings are the result of the storage in the muscles of toxins resulting from inappropriate dynamics (or "negative karma" as described in Chapter 3, Note 8). If this were true, the use of psychedelics would be an excellent way to clear this up. Consequently if the subject were willing to confront the uncomfortable feelings and stay with them, they would be resolved and it would be possible to enter an enjoyable state with 2C-B.

We decided to test this hypothesis; we asked those who had uncomfortable 2C-B experiences if they were willing to have additional experiences, confront their feelings, and seek resolution. In almost every case when the subject was willing to participate in such a program, within two or three additional sessions he/she became free of the body load and was able to achieve an enjoyable experience.

In the case of one couple, the body load each of them was carrying was so great that it was just too uncomfortable to go through the experience. When it didn't clear up in two tries, they didn't wish to carry the experiment any further. For those that did continue, they were gratified to experience the very special place that 2C-B makes available.

We were so intrigued with the properties of 2C-B that we worked with it almost exclusively for about a year. Another aspect we were very much interested in was the effectiveness of 2C-B following the initial ingestion of MDMA. Taking the MDMA first cleared up much of the body load problem, and paved the way to a much smoother 2C-B experience.

With this combination we ran into a new problem. We heard reports that MDMA and 2C-B were antagonistic, so supplementing with 2C-B canceled out the effects of both. We found this to be somewhat true. The solution that we and others found was to give the MDMA plenty of time to wear off before ingesting the 2C-B. We found that an adequate time was two to three hours. So taking 2C-B three hours after the last ingestion of MDMA (either the original dose or the supplement taken 1-1/2 hours later) led to a fruitful and enjoyable 2C-B experience.

Here are some excerpts from our trials. It is difficult to select from the large number of reports, as in almost every case the experiences are euphoric, uniformly rewarding, and instill awe at the grandeur of creation and the magnificence we are as human beings. I have chosen examples to illustrate the development of our knowledge, and some of the more outstanding events that transpired.

### *An Early Experience*

Jean and I start with 120 m.g. of MDMA. It is a marvelous experience with the usual effects – rejuvenation, youthfulness of skin, aliveness, bliss, bright colors. Looking into our optically ground mirror, we are each pleased with what we see – a good person to know; radiant, alive, lovable.

One hour 26 minutes later, we each take 2C-B: Jean 16 m.g., I take 20 m.g. As it comes on, I feel more expansive. Jean notices no difference from the MDMA state. We become quiet and listen to music. Outdoors the mountains are exquisite, resplendent with radiant light. The clouds are unusually beautiful with a softness and tenderness not encountered with other substances. At times things become very bright. I feel close to a deep level of love, but do not break completely through. The experience is not as profound as some.

Listening to music is very compelling. Jean has never responded so completely. I find the 2C-B more opening than MDMA; it is easier to contemplate a variety of subjects. The price for me is a diminution of the deep bliss and sense of wholeness. Outdoors it is easy to get absorbed in plants, the details of nature. I am swept away by a beautiful, transcendent feeling.

Late in the afternoon I note a change in the character of the experience. Earlier I felt that using volition, like consciously turning on love, was followed by an inner emptiness. During the descent I find volition helpful in changing the character of the experience. I can move to a higher level and feel bliss and love, which drains away inner tensions and discomforts. [From subsequent training in meditation, I surmise that I "built up merit", or having cleared away some inner obstacles, I was freer and had more energy to direct volition. At the time of this experience I preferred not to deal with the uncomfortable feelings that were surfacing.]

In late afternoon I went for my mile run. The first half was very difficult. But the body responded and the second half of the run was blissful, leaving all tensions behind. Lovemaking that night was exquisite.

The days following the experience were the best part. This is quite different than with other substances. Despite the experience not being particularly outstanding in profundity, there developed a feeling of inner strength and stability as though important interior changes had been achieved.

2C-B yields a very benign feeling and deep euphoria that seems quite special. It feels very friendly, and makes all the world appear friendly. Two days after my body feels light and cleansed. I have an eagerness to accomplish things, and experience a marvelous inner peace. In the evening, awaiting the arrival of company, while looking at the mountains and listening to music, I move into an elevated experience as profound as any during the journey itself. It is an even better feeling, as there is no inner tension or feeling of having taken a drug.

We had received information that when following MDMA with 2C-B, there was a tendency for the two drugs to cancel each other. So in the following experience, three months later than the one reported above, we purposely left a longer time interval between the ingestion of the drugs.

Jean and I take 120 m.g. of MDMA. We have our usual joyful experience. We realize that we need to do this, just the two of us, more often. We take a 40 m.g. supplement at 1-1/2 hours. We clear up many things in our relationship.

We purposefully wait 2-1/2 hours before taking 2C-B. Jean takes 16 m.g., the same as before; I take 25 m.g. Jean reports that the MDMA and 2C-B experience are all one. Then she notices that the 2C-B enhances taste; her mouth is more alive. Things separate out more. The experience continues to gather momentum. There is a gentleness, softness, subtlety to 2C-B. I feel that it will not be abused, as you have to learn how to turn it on. Otherwise you might not find much.

As we walk outside everything becomes intensely bright with brilliant colors. We enjoy the breeze, the clouds, the vistas of the mountains. The more we pay attention, the more magnificent it is. It doesn't have the intensity and clarity of LSD, but offers much more tenderness and inner wholeness. The intensity of the experience continues to develop for two full hours, at which point it is very potent. We find lovemaking exceptional, bringing closeness and fulfillment without orgasm.

Afterwards, sitting on the deck, it is most enjoyable to simply observe the sky, the clouds, and the mountains. Being still and letting go heightens the joy. There is a strong sense of Presence, not as intense as with LSD but in some ways warmer and more meaningful. All senses are turned on, which brings delight to eating and enjoying music.

The aftermath of this experience was the best thus far. The following day there is an all-pervading feeling of gentleness, kindness, and inner meaning. Inwardly I feel strong and solid, like it isn't going to go away, as the LSD exalted feeling sometimes feels. I feel a powerful change. Three days later I still feel it deeply, with much inner strength. A drive to a neighboring town two days after the experience is like a continuation of the session, with enhanced colors, beauty, and that pervading feeling of softness and gentleness. The third night I am still feeling +1 (see rating scale in Appendix II).

Supplementing with 2C-B certainly dispels the lethargy that tends to develop following MDMA alone. This combination, with time between ingestions, is excellent. The relationship between Jean and me has greatly improved, with real closeness, tenderness, and understanding. We are holding onto it better than after any previous experience.

Another trial: Jean, on 120 m.g. of MDMA followed by 20 m.g. of 2C-B at 2 hours. For the first time she becomes her spirit. Now she knows what everyone is writing about. What utter exaltation, peace, sense of infinity and eternity! She knows she will be all right no matter what happens to this planet.

### *With Other Couples*

a. 120 m.g. of MDMA followed by 40 m.g. supplement, followed by 2C-B: Jean 20 m.g.; Myron 25 m.g.; couple 30 m.g. each. Jean feels she has a bit too much; it became jangling, confusing, more like LSD. She enjoys the group very much. The couple felt that the 2C-B is more centering than LSD and like the feeling of inner wholeness. They feel it permits resolving more of what is going on in your life; it addresses more where you live. But it did not have the profound opening of the center produced by MDMA. After three days together we all felt centered, strong, relaxed, and with all of our problems resolved.

b. *Sabrina and Weldon.* Weldon is a good friend we have been working with for several months. He is deeply interested in spirituality, and committed to personal growth. He is a very complex person and has some serious emotional disturbances. We agreed to a series of six MDMA sessions with him. Although there was much learning, he was very subject to upheavals from his unconscious, which manifested in a great variety of imagery and disturbing thoughts and feelings. Sabrina is an attractive girl of 36. She had numerous psychedelic experiences in her younger days, but has not explored for several years. She is anxious to try the new substances. Weldon hopes that the addition of 2C-B and the support of his girl friend will yield greater progress.

We take 120 m.g. of MDMA, followed by 2C-B: Weldon 12 m.g. (because of his very unusual sensitivity), Sabrina 18 m.g., Jean and I 20 m.g. Sabrina lights up dramatically with MDMA, becoming a happy young girl, full of life and spirit. She feels the 2C-B a continuation of the MDMA experience.

Under the 2C-B, Weldon develops a feeling of well-being. He is able to pass through and discard the kinds of disturbances that have bothered him in past sessions. He feels stronger, and that he has made much progress. The feeling of solidity and euphoria grow throughout the day. We experience exceptionally close bonding, and all have a marvelous time. Sabrina dances beautifully to Japanese music; we enjoy musical selections. That evening an excellent recording of Christmas music drives home deeply the experience of Christ Consciousness and what it means for the world.

### *Reincarnation*

Many experience under the influence of psychedelics what appears to be past lifetimes. Whether these are actual or the mind's symbolic way of portraying dynamics is difficult to prove. To the one who experiences them they seem very real, as in the second session reported below.

There are a number of therapists who practice Past Lives Therapy. The premise is that the patient's problems arise from an event in a previous lifetime. Even though I am personally convinced that reincarnation is real, and have gathered data for other writing which makes a strong case for it, I prefer to hold an open mind and be aware of alternate interpretations of experience.

The human mind is enormously creative, and under appropriate circumstances can create intriguing, sharply detailed events that carry powerful feelings of authenticity. Research with hypnotized subjects reveals how readily good subjects may be suggested into a particular time and place, and begin to describe people, events, costumes, and environments appropriate to that time and place.

Whether or not Past Life therapists are able to get their clients to actually experience past lives, I have always thought that it is a very useful mechanism. This is because it allows the client to search his/her unconscious for the source of the problem without having the burden of responsibility for acts in this lifetime. Once the problem surfaces and is acknowledged as having occurred in the past, it is easier for the client to deal with it. When resolved, then the implications for this lifetime can be addressed.

So regardless of the authenticity of past lifetime events, two experiences described below illustrate how they may surface in a psychedelic experience:

> a. On 120 m.g. of MDMA followed by a 40 m.g. supplement, then 30 m.g. of 2C-B: The male subject feels he has experienced a previous lifetime. He reviewed the akashic records[2] to see where he had gotten off the path to enlightenment. He felt there were three lifetimes where he might have made it, but didn't. They were all similar, and he failed in the same way each time. This was by trying to be the good guy, bringing in light and love. But he had never been strong enough to prevent being overcome by evil-doers. So he felt betrayed. Now he is afraid to expose his feelings as they will be used against him. He must be wary of people.

b. *Another experience involving past lifetimes*. Experiences with sacramental substances can take many different turns. The combination of a special group of people, and a particular agreed upon direction, can strongly influence the nature of the experience and the outcomes. This journey is with a person well experienced in using sacramental substances, and highly motivated in a spiritual direction.

> We start with 120 m.g. each of MDMA. I am suddenly hit very hard, going into instant euphoria. It's my most sudden takeoff to date. We agree to an interior experience, and the three of us – Jean, our friend, and I – lie side by side on a bed, listening to Kitaro's Silk Road. This is my first interior journey with MDMA, a process which I find very much intensifies the experience. It is outstanding, the music exquisite, and we have profound, elated feelings. Compared to the usual experience, it is more intense and compelling. However, it doesn't last as long, as this process seems to "use up" the substance. In an hour I feel I am coming down, though I feel at peace.
>
> We take 2C-B two hours later, Jean 20 m.g., our friend and I 25 m.g. We continue to listen to music. The experience reaches the peak obtained with the MDMA, and then goes even deeper. I see the most beautiful visuals I have ever seen with 2C-B – they have a softness and gentleness characteristic of this

material. Letting go to the experience is a superb feeling, regardless of the content. At times I go through pain, but it doesn't matter. I simply accept it as part of the flow. The music gets more and more compelling.

Suddenly I am overcome with deep, intense anger. I am so angry that killing means nothing. I experience myself as as brutal captain, like Genghis Khan, leading hordes on horses and killing people right and left. The depth of my anger makes it easy to reach out and kill. There is even satisfaction in destroying others. I laugh contemptuously at pain and death as I urge my men on. My anger is finally spent; then I see that the life I am now leading is to help atone for this past behavior.

I wonder about forgiveness; I see that even killers are forgiven if they can forgive themselves. This makes me think of Jesus dying on the cross to forgive our sins. It works if we can accept it in the depth of our being. Anything at all that we can use to get us to realize we are forgiven helps achieve forgiveness. These realizations make me feel much kinder toward Fundamentalist Christians.

I wonder if I would die for others. I feel an enormous love for God. The only thing to do is love and live the truth when it is appropriate. If we are killed for the truth it's all right, since we are indestructible and will simply appear again in another body.

At this time I feel myself slipping easily out of one lifetime into another, in a succession of reincarnations. As I focus on what is happening, it appears that the change-points are the most difficult, especially the birth process. I seem to have a difficult time with getting born. I postulate an easy birth and things get better.

By mid-afternoon the music is superbly outstanding. Each instrument stands out clearly in magnificent harmony and melody. Love, beauty, euphoria overcome us all. I am feeling exquisite freedom and ecstasy, when all of a sudden I realize I have died!

I laugh as I realize it is exactly as Jacob has described death. Jacob is an outstanding psychedelic therapist who has monitored over three thousand experiences. He claims that it is not a real death if you are trying to die and observe the process. With real death, you don't know you are dying until you are suddenly aware that you have died.

Now it is clear that we can never die because we are eternal; we always have been and always will be. Death is an illusion. What dies is the pile of garbage from the past that I have been dearly holding onto. As I let this go, I can be completely here and now in the moment; this is being utterly alive. Words cannot describe the joy of this experience, or how marvelous it is to be free to flow with the music and whatever develops.

Our friend is far, far out, experiencing himself as pure spirit. To talk, he reports that he has to come down through levels to get back to the viewpoint of his body. His mind is crystal clear and his perceptions extremely sensitive.

As the experience draws to an end, I have a clear, profound view of honesty. I see more clearly than ever before how easy it is, after such experiences, to let the perception of who we really are fuzz up and return to old ways of perceiving, judging, and evaluating.

This was an exceptionally outstanding experience, for which we were all truly grateful.

## *Benefit of Therapists*

One important experience Jean and I shared with MDMA followed by 2C-B was with two young, very competent therapists. It was an outstanding experience, in which all participants fully realized the major attributes of these two substances. Our journey was greatly enhanced by the outstanding qualities of these therapists as persons and as skilled professionals. Because of their experience, the conduct of our session followed some fresh approaches. Here are some of the ways:

Chris and Kay strongly affirm and express the good qualities they perceive in each of us. We feel their honesty, sincerity, and love. They also frankly talk in a loving way about possible limitations they see in us. They are quite helpful and supportive in helping us find improved ways of relating.

They comment on my way of being a loner and functioning by myself; Jean's way of working alone in the kitchen that makes it difficult for others to help. They are aware of unresolved areas within us, and keep us focused on it with questions. They support us with love and energy enhanced by touching, and are not satisfied until we break through to the essence of the difficulty.

In keeping with the general development of the experience, we each in turn became the center of group attention until there is a breakthrough or new realization. The height of the experience for Jean and me comes when we realize how much we shut each other out and need to affirm each other.

Chris states that there is a part of our partner that our unconscious recognized in choosing him/her for a mate. He and Kay have each made a commitment to affirm that part. When Kay asks Jean about her commitment to me, it becomes apparent that she has none, which was an extremely painful blow to me, to the extent that I cry deeply. This in turn opens a great flow of love between Jean and me.

As we progress it becomes clear that the experience mounts in intensity as each person is real and creative; playing an old tape breaks the magic and progression. As we deepen and enrich communication, it results in an enormous flow of love and intimate closeness.

I learn in a very concrete way how wonderful it is to share a problem openly and honestly and get the love and support of the group rather than trying to work it through alone. And how important it is when someone is transmitting to make sure the message is really received.

Most of my life I have felt it quite sufficient to rely on the Inner Teacher, especially with the greater access provided by a good sacrament. But the Inner Teacher can work through many instruments, as was so aptly demonstrated in this experience. Wise, knowledgeable companions are an enormous asset on sacramental journeys.

### Chapter 4 Notes

1. Shulgin, A. T. & Shulgin, A. *PIHKAL, A Chemical Love Story*. Berkeley, California: Transform Press, 1991, pp. 503-6.
2. Akashic Records. There are a number of esoteric disciplines that incorporate a concept of Universal Mind, somewhat along the lines of Carl Jung's Collective Unconscious. It is held that all thoughts and all actions that have ever taken place exist in this Universal Mind, and comprise the Akashic Records. Thus should one develop

the ability to enter Universal Mind with freedom, these records are considered to be available and can be consulted. Any event that has ever transpired could be recalled and examined. In determining the validity of such observations, it is well to heed the warning of contemplative orders, who point out the difficulty of determining the difference between true inspiration and active imagination. See Appendix IV, Note 1.

# Chapter 5
# Other New Compounds

A large number of compounds have been discovered which are psychoactive. Jean and I have had the opportunity to try several of them, and found a few that were outstanding in their characteristics and warranted further attention. We describe below some of the results on compounds with which we had the most experience, as well as some that we liked but did not have the opportunity to investigate further.

## *MEM*

My first trial of MEM, code name for 2,5-dimethoxy-4-ethoxyamphetamine,[1] was not overly impressive. It revealed the characteristics of a good psychedelic, but demonstrated nothing to indicate an advantage over a number of other good compounds. We did find, however, that it had outstanding attributes when preceded by MDMA.

The first trial of MDMA followed by MEM was with a group and was quite successful. It was the most enjoyable experience so far with this particular group. For the first time I felt no discontinuity in the transition from MDMA to the second substance. There followed a most delightful afternoon of intimate sharing, good communication, hilarity, and deep appreciation of one another. The experience continued until midnight. Most important, the changes involving inner strength, solidarity, and peace carried on much longer than any previous experience.

With this very moving result, we were anxious to continue investigating this combination. We soon repeated the experience, just Jean and I. Again I found it an uninterrupted continuation of the MDMA experience. We had our most detailed discussion to date, clarifying a lot of our history and feelings, ever growing closer. We found that MEM has great power, continuing without letup for hours, well into the night (we started at ten a.m.). We had good physical control, and could do whatever we wished in terms of tasks. Yet the experience was intense. When we retired, we grew into a closeness never before experienced, a superb encounter that united our inner beings.

With this data, we wished to expand our knowledge of this combination with other subjects. Several cases are reported below.

### *An Occluded Case*

Ken is a 28 year old musician, earning his living as a computer operator in a small business firm. He has had MDMA three times with his guide, who joins us now.

He and the guide take 130 m.g. of MDMA followed by a supplement of 45 m.g. Three hours after the start we all take 20 m.g. of MEM. Two hours later Ken and I take 10 m.g. more, as I find the going very heavy. [Additional chemical is required to overcome heavy resistance or blockages.]

We make a very close and productive group. Ken is very honest, and likes candid, intimate discussion. As we share with each other, we are drawn very close. We make the transition to MEM with no loss of the euphoric and centering MDMA feeling.

Our discussion continues unabated through the afternoon and evening, pushed by a powerful drive from the MEM. It is the most intense, continuing discussion I have participated in. We all learn a great deal from each other and continue to draw closer. A major point of the discussion is whether or not Ken should drop his rather pedestrian job to concentrate on his music.

That night I am very restless, as I feel we failed to reach resolution, despite the power and drive of the substance. Ken does not reach his deep inner feelings, and I feel a heavy wall between us. The following morning I see Ken as a very sensitive person struggling to come to terms with his inner self; he needs much time and support. On a walk the next morning we have excellent, free communication, and the wall I feel dissolves. We both feel much power.

Jean and I believe this combination has enormous impact with unusual strength. It is long lasting, and keeps one working away at his/her difficulties. Ken was carrying a heavy psychic burden, and succeeded in freeing himself from much of it.

### *Resolving a Marriage*

Liz is a 26 year old girl, very attractive, outgoing and full of spunk. She is in an unfortunate marriage, where the partners are quite different and have a difficult time appreciating each other. Liz has strayed from the path and now realizes it will not work out. But does she want to continue in her present marriage?

We have several days of good, open discussion, in which Liz reviews her feelings and options. She asks for this experience to reach and know her deeper feelings.

We all take 120 m.g. of MDMA, and it exhibits its usual positive effects. 1-2/3 hours later we take 20 m.g. of MEM. The transition to MEM is smooth except for Liz, who has a lot of discomfort. She feels her problem is making her whole body uncomfortable. She is achy, has a headache and back pain. She struggles with this all day, not feeling any resolution and not feeling like talking. She is slowly working things out. She feels quite tired most of the day, which affects Jean and me. It is a hard working day.

While Liz is working, I take her 2-1/2 year old son for a walk. He is a great teacher. I find him remarkably bright and in tune. He knows exactly when I divert my attention from him, and when I am not completely truthful with him. He soaks up information, new words, and new procedures like a hungry sponge, as long as I give him my complete attention.

I have an outstanding day, seeing Jean's celestial beauty and experiencing the indescribable essence of female. The driving power of the MEM lasts all night. To be comfortable, I have to keep focusing the power outward, flowing love into situations, to people I know, to healing the world. This is extremely cleansing and uplifting. I awake the following morning feeling elated, body cleansed and in a very sound, stable place.

I am concerned that Liz might have been pushed too hard by this combination. She awoke with a bad cold and was tired. She slept in. When she arose she felt she had resolved the situation, and wanted to continue the marriage if her partner agreed. She is glad for the experience and found it helpful.

Two days later, Liz has well integrated this experience. She feels very good and has high resolve. She reported that she knew all the time what the outcome would be, but had to clear away the feelings of anger, disappointment, and pain until her true feelings could come in strongly. She abandoned thinking to simply letting go of her feelings and letting them work through. Talking to her husband on the phone, when he reported that he was eager to have her back, all the achiness in her body suddenly ceased.

Jean and I both felt a new power and confidence in Liz, like a quantum leap forward.

The marriage didn't last; it broke up six months later. But Liz had found excellent strength to deal with all the contingencies. Two years later she found a much more compatible mate. They are living together happily, and have three more children between them.

. . . . . . .

After the two above experiences, I wrote to friends describing my evaluation of this combination:

At this point, I feel that the MDMA-MEM combination is the most powerful therapeutic combination that we have. Compared to the MDMA–2C-B combination, which we also hold in excellent regard, the MEM combination has a smoother transition into the second substance, so that it is more of a continuation of the MDMA state. The MEM is more centering, like MDMA, which makes it easy to work with and yet permits normal functioning on physical tasks. There seem to be less side-avenues and body effects than with 2C-B. There is a powerful push from the substance which keeps one working in a positive direction for a number of hours.

A possible drawback is that it may push people into areas for which they are not ready. Consequently subjects should be well motivated to address their problems if they wish to employ this combination.

While the body feels good and cleansed afterward, a lot of work has been done and there is quite a drain on the body. Recovery of full energy may take several days.

## *Sabrina*

Sabrina, our beloved adopted daughter, is moving out of the area to a new location where we will most likely seldom see her. In her new location, she will be able to conduct her practice as a midwife with proper medical supervision. We are having one last experience together to give her a chance to evaluate the new combination we feel is so effective.

Jean, Sabrina, and I take 120 m.g. of MDMA. We have preceded this two hours earlier with a 600 m.g. capsule of potassium chloride (Micro-K Extencaps) which we have found reduces the dehydration effects of MDMA and results in more comfortable body feelings. We quickly move into a beautiful, loving experience with much warmth and closeness. We walk to the spot where Sabrina had once erected a teepee, and then to the sweat lodge she had constructed. Both of these are very important to the Native American Indian work to which Sabrina feels called. It is very sad and beautiful as we recount our outstanding times together, and the pain of our separating. But we know she moves on into a new, productive, adventurous life, and we accept it with grace.

An hour and a half later, Sabrina takes 20 m.g. of MEM, Jean and I 15 m.g. each. There is a very smooth transition into the MEM experience. In about 15 minutes, we begin to feel more power and openness. We stay in good communication and closeness. We cannot believe it when we observe that two hours have gone by.

An hour later we take another capsule of potassium chloride. Still another hour later, I feel very dehydrated and take a third capsule, which resolves the problem.

We have a wonderful afternoon, but no profound heights. In the late afternoon Sabrina is experiencing back pains and a headache. She decides to go to a neighbor to take a hot-tub.

I suggest that before she leaves, we try Gendlin's focusing procedure (see Chapter 4, Note 9) for her bodily discomforts. She agrees.

She lies down on the couch and goes into it immediately. I feel strongly guided; the procedure flows easily. I feel much pain in Sabrina. The handles she chooses are words like pain, pressure, dark, block, hold; she moves through them with little resistance. At the end of forty-five minutes I wonder if she has accomplished enough. She reports that she is continually uncovering deeper layers, so we proceed.

Suddenly the word "pierce" comes, and she moves into a spontaneous experience. She feels that she is in a past life, and is fleeing with her people from the enemy. She feels that she is masculine, and is either their shaman or their leader.

She feels very tired, and that her work is done and that it is time to go. She stands between her people and the enemy, and "calls the lance", which strikes her in the neck. Her people pull her and drag her with them. She cries, "No, no!" feeling deeply that they don't understand, that it is her time to go, and to leave her alone. They finally comprehend and leave her to die, which is a great release.

She then goes through a long, dark tunnel, continually asking, "Why is there so much pain?" She sees some light in a circle around the opening of the tunnel; here there is peace. I can feel her resistance dissolving, and the peace and exultation move in.

She experiences the very deep pain she feels with her father, being completely misunderstood and isolated. Because her father rejected her, she rejected her father. Now she sees this is senseless revenge, bringing much, much pain to them both. She gains deep insight and understanding of their relationship.

Next she finds that it is really true, the body can handle the vast energy from above. One doesn't have to leave the body and go to another level for this vitality. But to handle this prodigious energy, one must not let the body dictate, but must direct the energy properly.

Sabrina has an enormous release with great peace and euphoria, which invades us all. I feel all of my own load drop as Sabrina moves into this experience of exultation. A profound understanding passes between Sabrina and me. I feel that at last she truly sees herself and me. She expresses that she has felt me with her all the way. She says, "Midwives need midwives", which moves me to tears.

From my standpoint, I simply sat quietly, focusing my energy without conceptual thought. As she went through the tunnel, I felt that she needed to learn to shift her focus from pain to peace. I held my focus on peace, and the peace and exultation grew enormously as she broke through. I have no way of knowing whether my silent focusing helped her steer in this direction, or whether the increase in peace that I felt simply resulted from her reaching this level. In any event, both Jean and I were lifted to high levels of exultation. [My current understanding, a number of years after this experience, is that the bonding becomes so great in these experiences that we are very likely co-experiencing strong feelings.]

Following her breakthroughs, Sabrina looks very young. Her back pains are gone, and there is an enormous bond among the three of us. She still has some headache, for which she takes tylenol. We get further release of deep feelings through dancing to high energy dance music.

We retire with an enormous feeling of accomplishment. We can think of no better way to help Sabrina embark on her new journey.

## *2C-T-2*

2C-T-2, code name for 2,5-dimethoxy-4-ethylthiophenethylamineh[2], is one of the best general purpose psychedelics we have run across. It is effective over a dose range of 12 to 30 m.g. We have occasionally used it at lower doses, 8 to 10 m.g., for the purpose of monitoring others taking MDMA, as mentioned in Chapter 3.

We found it to be an excellent general purpose work horse. It retains some of the euphoric centering qualities of MDMA, which make it pleasant to work with. At the same time, it provides considerably more opening, similar to the more powerful psychedelics such as LSD, without the propensity of the latter to drop one into disturbing pools of repressed feelings. This permits exploring a wide range of levels of thought and inner feelings. It is a long acting substance which can take up an entire day. The plateau at peak lasts for a good five hours, giving one plenty of time to work and enjoy.

There is not the driving push from the drug that the classic psychedelics provide, so that one retains considerably more volition. Yet there is sufficient drive to explore any area that is truly desired, from one's own feelings to interpersonal relationships to the nature of the cosmos. Motivation is the key. With practice the earnest seeker can use 2C-T-2 to investigate whatever area of consciousness interests her/him. And for the most part, it is a comfortable, enjoyable vehicle with which to do the exploring.

Our first experience of 2C-T-2 was with a group of close friends. I take 14 m.g., Jean 12 m.g. The drug is quite gradual in its onset, taking about two hours to reach full intensity.

> As the intensity develops, I develop some of my entry-type discomfort. Fortunately after an hour or so, this dissipates and I enter into a stage of enjoyment. This is facilitated by the bantering and good will of the group. We all reach a good space, charged with energy. This leads to the most enjoyable interchange I have experienced with this group up to this date. We find that the chemical has considerably heightened our sense of humor and creativeness to have fun. We also have insightful discussions. We find it difficult to break up before midnight.
>
> This experience left me quite whole and well-centered. The only thing missing is what I call the spiritual element, or my feeling the presence of God. Yet driving home four days later I had profound spiritual realizations.

Our first replication of 2C-T-2 without the group came several months later, with the same dosage:

> We move into the experience progressing alternatively between positive and negative feelings. We are able to discuss our feelings with each other more freely than ever before. We are both aware of our deep anger with each other, and are able to express it without rancor. Jean feels smothered by me, and I see clearly how I do this.
>
> I discover within myself a feeling of being "left out", and how painful this is. I am driven to many useless devices to avoid this pain. As I look at myself through the eyes of my friends, I find no qualities that would make them seek my company. I am able to see this with detachment and humor, and am able to laugh at my always striving to be front and center. I try 'feeling wanted' on for size, and this helps me feel better.
>
> We discuss freedom, and the importance of giving it to each other. This makes me feel a painful loneliness, but is a worthwhile price to pay for granting freedom. I feel that God is very lonely in extending freedom to His people. But He would never violate the personal freedom of others to escape loneliness. He greatly appreciates those who recognize and acknowledge Him. [I realize that the concept that God can be lonely may violate some people's ideas of God. But as I have deepened my personal relationship with God over the years, and comprehend more than ever the vastness of the Mystery that we cannot fathom, I still hold to this view. I personally cherish my anthropomorphic view of God. While this is a very narrow aspect of a vast reality, it is still personally very meaningful to me. This position has at times helped me through some very rough places, as these reports indicate.]
>
> Music is powerful, and I reach a magnificent height in which I experience the Supreme Female. She is indescribable beautiful, exquisitely loving, sensitive, tender, nourishing; it is worth life itself to be even momentarily in a ray of this magnificent Presence. I move higher to achieve complete union with this Presence. I feel fear because I am alone, and I'm afraid that without the support and relationship of others, I will move into a private, narrow world and be totally unconcerned for others. At this moment Jean enters the room! I reach heights of love and beauty, totally discharging any uncomfortable feelings.
>
> Despite this, another wave of anger comes over me at the excruciating pain of being rejected. I see that I am rejecting Jean in many ways. The anger continues to grow, until I decide to turn the experience around by consciously creating love. To do this I find I must be very gentle, not forcing it, but allowing the love to build up. This incorporates the principals I had discovered in the

Supreme Female. This brought back all the marvelous feelings of joy, beauty, and transcendence I had experienced before.

This experience was remarkably rejuvenating, and felt like a new lease on life. Here is another experience with a young couple who were undergoing considerable difficulty in their relationship. Joyce and Vern have lived together for five years. They have shared several sacramental journeys, with real growth in understanding. Vern has a very lucrative business installing concrete footings and foundations, but his body is giving out on him, so that he is in constant stress and pain.

Joyce is fed up with living in an incomplete house, and with what she describes as Vern's rigidity, not acknowledging her, being totally immersed in himself and his work, and carrying such a huge burden of heaviness that she no longer enjoys being around him. She openly discusses leaving him.

We have a long, exploratory discussion to determine whether there is any point in having an experience. Joyce does not want to leave harboring so much resentment and wants to find love for herself and Vern. Vern wishes to drop his heavy burdens and find how to enter a new vocation of finishing wood work, which he very much loves.

We all take 2C-T-2, Joyce and Vern 14 m.g. each, Jean and I 12 m.g. The intensity increases steadily for three hours. We have easy conversation, covering many aspects of the dynamics of life. Joyce is sharp, alert, and clear-headed, a joy to talk with. Vern is quiet, pleasant, strong, likable, and hard-working. It is clear he is well over his head, both in the relationship and in the projects he is trying to complete without adequate time.

At one point we lie down with our heads touching, and listen to a tape. Both have participated in Indian ceremonies, so we choose *Sounds of the Shaman.* It is a powerful tape of a highly developed American Indian Shaman producing a variety of intense sounds – long, pronounced deep breathing, rattles, bird cries, evocations. These sounds are created to facilitate moving into unfamiliar states of awareness. It causes Joyce to confront her fears, and she finds herself proceeding from the position of a frightened mouse to an eagle, from the untrusting coyote to trust.

The rest of the day goes beautifully, with excellent communication, clear insights, and a powerful euphoria growing in all of us. We experience love, trust and gratitude for the wonder and beauty of life. Joyce and Vern reach a point where they feel good being together; they have cleared up a great deal of negative material within themselves. They talk openly and honestly, with much greater understanding of each other. Joyce finds many fine qualities in Vern she had been unwilling to see before.

Vern feels that he has dropped a heavy load, and can approach his tasks at home with renewed energy, fresh attitudes and understanding. He now feels that the stress of their deteriorating relationship may be partially responsible for his body problems. He finds that he is enjoying concrete work more than he had realized. However, he does want to get out of this hard physical labor.

They left the next day much happier, freer, and with a great deal more understanding and willingness to confront their situation. Joyce is not sure if she will stay, but at least she will leave knowing that she loves Vern.

Jean and I both had an excellent experience. We learned to surmount our own personal concerns and thereby be better companions for others struggling with problems. Joyce found 2C-T-2 excellent to work with. It allowed her to look into the dark places without pushing her. She knew she had the choice to turn away if she wished, but her honesty compelled her to get as much as possible from the experience.

Continued use of 2C-T-2 revealed many valuable properties. We gained a great deal of experience with this substance personally, and with a number of subjects. A more formal investigation was conducted with the first time use of 40 subjects, and is reported in the reference of Chapter 4, Note 2.

## *2C-T-7*

2C-T-7, code name for 2,5-dimethoxy-4-(n)-propylthiophenethylamine[3], is another one of the outstanding phenethylamine compounds. In many respects it is very similar to 2C-T-2. It has the same dose range, although there have been occasions where 10 m.g was quite powerful and adequate. It takes about two hours to reach full intensity, has a broad, approximately five hour plateau of full activity, and has a long, gradual descent. There is evidence that it is even more euphoric than 2C-T-2. Several of our subjects who experienced dark regions with 2C-T-2 discovered 2C-T-7 to be continually enjoyable. Here is the report of our first trial with 2C-T-7:

> We each start with 12 m.g. Not much is happening, so an hour and a half later, Jean takes an additional 3 m.g. and I add 8 m.g. I spend most of the day releasing to my Inner Teacher. I clear up a deep charge of loneliness. Later I find it satisfying to respond immediately to inner impulses without squelching them. I do some neglected repair work on power lines feeding our pump house. Using a hacksaw, I learn how tense and compulsive I am, and how much better things work by relaxing and letting the universe cooperate.
>
> Later, relaxing on the deck, my thinking is free and clear. My previous chore demonstrated the power of focusing the mind. I now focus on love, with most rewarding results. Vestiges of discomfort clear up. I see the great value of holding love in the face of diversity. I get a powerful insight: let any feeling of discomfort remind me of the wonder, beauty, and bountifulness of the universe. This works much better than my habitual response, which is to wonder what is wrong.
>
> I discover my strong desire for POWER, and how wonderful it feels to permit it to course through my being. I have worked hard to hide this realization from myself. As I share this with Jean, she says "Of course!" as if to say, what else is new? "Power is useful, but it must always be used with love."
>
> I see I still hold restrictions on Jean. As I relinquish them, I can freely explore various dimensions of her being. This is enormously rewarding. We agree to drop our restrictions on each other and be true friends.
>
> I get the clearest realization yet of how everything I look at is part of me. I have no sense of self-boundary. Everything exists to help us if we can just let it in. Wonder and beauty are everywhere. I don't need to manipulate anything; just letting things be is ultimate satisfaction.

This experience relieved me of much burden I was carrying, permitting me to function more effectively. I am much more able to stay focused on my writing. I have lost my sense of impatience while doing menial tasks. Also, some arthritis in my thumb that was threatening to become chronic disappeared. I feel this is an excellent substance, very clear, very permissive, and easier on the body than 2C-T-2.

A month later:

> Jean takes 18 m.g. of 2C-T-7; I take 20 m.g. Jean becomes very intoxicated, very much enjoying the experience. We have excellent communication, sharing our resentments of each other and what we wish of our partner that we have not been receiving. We find that we each have withheld many private thoughts from each other. Our discussion clears up many areas of misunderstanding, but most importantly, yields a marvelous feeling of inner freedom. I discover that a lot of the psychic burden I carry is "withholds" – things I think and feel but don't verbalize. Declaring what is on my mind produces a wonderful sense of freedom.
>
> We reach an intensity of enjoyment beyond what we have previously experienced together. We deeply feel our love for each other, and greatly appreciate the enchantment of our surroundings. The beauty grows with focused appreciation. I find the secret is "to let God live"; to allow His presence at all times in whatever we are doing. Jean and I commit ourselves to maintaining this outstanding space of love and clear communication.

Despite the closeness developed in these experiences, difficulties arose in Jean's and my relationship. Continued work exposed ever deeper layers of anger and self-hatred, which we projected on each other. Jean, never deeply involved in self-awareness, was confronted with a variety of new feelings. And despite my becoming more loving, my improved perceptions resulted in me becoming more critical and frustrated. I also believed that I had done all that I could to resolve my own feelings, and that I could not find comfort unless Jean resolved her resentments, which seemed unlikely.

We reached a breaking point and decided to part. But we had planned to attend a weekend retreat at Sky High Ranch, and agreed to complete this before any final decisions. As it turned out, we both received a good deal of valuable counseling there, which convinced us that our miserable feelings were of our own creation. This resulted in a decision to make our relationship work. The following experience followed shortly after this:

> Jean takes 18 m.g. of 2C-T-7, I take 20 m.g. We spend a good deal of time clarifying communication, agreeing on household procedures, reviewing our histories, discussing her mother and her dislike for me. Many things come to light, but Jean is very uncomfortable. There is a heavy weight between us.
>
> We listen to music, and we are carried away. I see we can open up to the universe, leave the gritty stuff behind, and look for the best of all possible worlds. This means seeing the highest in each other, acknowledging, supporting, and empowering each other.
>
> My experience completely turns around, and the heaviness evaporates into love. I see Jean totally differently. There is an infinite source of love to draw upon, and there is no such thing as tiredness. Energy and love are always available. The first commandment resounds through me, in its utter, full dimensions. I fully comprehend what it means to love God with *all* my heart and *all* my soul and *all* my strength and *all* my mind. It is mind-boggling, an incomprehensible love.
>
> I look around at the sky and the mountains, and ask to see what is the true nature of reality if I do absolutely nothing to influence it. A great euphoria begins to quietly build. I do nothing to encourage it, but simply keep observing.

An enormous power grows within, and everything is filled with light. I see that my concept of the Central Power Source is accurate. Focusing on this creates some tensions in my body. These have been formed by previous striving, and are now surfacing into awareness. As I observe the tensions and release them as with vipassana breath meditation, they dissipate. Everything flows together in the extraordinary space of pure, harmonious existence.

All the difficulties with Jean have evaporated, and we enjoy an outstanding closeness and harmony. I see her at times with a remarkable inner beauty shining forth, the manifestation of her Celestial nature, which simply melts me in love.

This experience cemented the change in our relationship. While it was not the end of our differences or our difficulties, it brought a determination on both of our parts to make our relationship work.

Jean and I reaped a great deal of personal benefit from 2C-T-7. We observed its use on numerous occasions with others, which confirmed our assessment of the value of this compound. The more formal study of 2C-T-2 described above included seven subjects who took 2C-T-7.

### *Limited Experience*

Of the remaining substances we have tried on a limited basis, there are a few that are worth mentioning because of their interesting potential. These are described below.

### *2C-T-21*

2C-T-21, code name for 2,5-dimethoxy-4-(2-fluoroethylthio)phenethylamine[4], is a very interesting substance, quite different from the other psychoactive drugs. In fact, it is not psychedelic, but a wonderful energizer. It raises mood and spirit, raises the energy level, increases wit and sense of humor, facilitates communication, and in general provides an excellent good time. All of this with no sacrifice in appetite. Most of the other active compounds tend to be anorectic during their active period. In short, it produces the state that most people are looking for when they drink alcohol, but without drunkenness or depressing any other faculties. There is no hangover, but instead a reasonable amount of bodily rejuvenation. So it is a laudable compound for group enjoyment when no serious work is intended.

Jean and I have enjoyed a number of excellent sessions with friends using this chemical. I was curious to see what the results would be when I took it alone:

I feel greater intensity than with the group. Looking inside, I find I can examine issues, and look at several. The most interesting is examining my concept of the Central Furnace. This is my understanding that the center of our being is our essence where life energy manifests, and it is through this life energy that we are connected to all others and the rest of creation. My experience is that as you approach this core, you discover a brilliant, penetrating, overpowering light of indescribable beauty. This is love itself, or God, residing at our central core. This is what I call the Central Furnace.

In this experience, I get a sense of it, and attempt to intensify it. As I do this, it seems to me that I simultaneously intensify Hell, as Heaven and Hell must stay in balance. So it is better to achieve some transcendent level that integrates them both.

But four days later, I have to revise my evaluation. I have a lasting feeling of a central, interior warmth within myself. This was produced by my willingness to concentrate on the Central Furnace for some time. Giving it my attention helped to bring it into reality.

Now I see no harm in doing this. In fact, it produced a considerable benefit. As I now understand it, if it is attempted out of one's willful determination, the result is as first described. Willfully attempting to create the positive automatically creates its counterpart, the negative. Now it seems clear that the proper procedure is to focus, or ask, and then let the development come from a deeper source within, which takes surrender. This clearly seems the way to become Co-Creator. [This ties in with my concept of being partners with God, a view that runs through most of my major experiences.]

2C-T-21 permits bending to some extent to individual exploration, but is far surpassed in this regard by many other compounds. Its most satisfying use appears to be in group situations as described above.

A word of caution: One experienced couple we know fell into a dark, frightening hole with this compound. They were convinced that it is toxic. It is extremely important to remember that when working with these substances, there is no such thing as a casual experiment. One must always have recourse to knowledge and skillful means, and always be prepared for unexpected eruptions of the unconscious mind. As far as I know, no one else has reported a similar difficulty with 2C-T-21.

## *2C-T-4*

2C-T-4, code name for 2,5-dimethoxy-4-(i)-propylthiophenethylamine[5], has characteristics quite similar to 2C-T-2 except that it is considerably longer acting. We have had it only twice, and our first experience with it was outstanding. We found it more benign than 2C-T-2, perhaps because lasting all day and evening, the intensity of the chemical grew more gradually and was easier to handle. We found it a superb way to put in a long day. Here is a report of our first trial:

Jean takes 8 m.g. and I take 9 m.g. of 2C-T-4. We have a marvelous ascent – clean, gentle, and smooth. Our perception is heightened, and conversation is easy. We enjoy talking over many things for which we ordinarily don't take time.

I spend a good deal of time exploring inside, which is very rewarding. It is easy to explore questions and find answers. I strike a deep loneliness, which resolves as my love for myself grows. I focus on self-love until I finally break free with a substantial appreciation of myself. This is most fulfilling.

The experience grows in intensity over a three hour period, and stays at the peak for many hours afterward. It becomes a complete, profound, and thorough exploration. This is a remarkable substance, allowing me to look anywhere and explore any chosen subject. Bodywise, it is clean and clear. The experience remains smooth and gentle. Even exploring uncomfortable areas, there is still a good feeling tone. I see clearly into my own functioning, relationships, the dynamics of people I focus on, and general philosophical truths.

I find it best to let go and simply flow with the experience, following wherever it takes me. This leads to a growing euphoria, a feeling of clearing out body residues, and often culminates in profound insight. Thinking continues to grow in clarity throughout the day, and visual perception is crystal clear. The scenery is outstanding. Closeness and understanding with Jean develop steadily during the day. It is a most enjoyable time together.

A major problem I work on is the sluggish feelings that arise from time to time. I find it best to simply ride them through. As the day develops, it becomes easier to change my feelings by changing the focus of my thoughts. A major lesson is honesty, to simply be what I am with all of my idiosyncrasies, and stop trying to make things different. I achieve an exceptional state of peace and contentment with myself and the way things are.

Dancing to high energy dance music uncovers a lot of new, intense feelings, leading to some of the most profound realizations of the day. I strike a profound dichotomy: on the one hand, everyone is God and can resolve their own burdens, so I don't have to do anything. On the other hand, I am Christ and only by my being willing to lift the burden of others can the world be helped. [This is somewhat like a high level realization I experienced sometime later with my friend Gil (see Chapter 11), that the highest state of all is caring with all of your might, while simultaneously not caring with all of your might. Whoever comprehends this is well along the path!]

I see there is nothing wrong with having high standards, as long as I apply them to myself. I profoundly see the equality of everyone, and my proper relationship to others.

Persons on tight time schedules will have a hard time working in the occasion for 2C-T-4. Jean and I like setting aside a day for an experience, and that being the case, it might as well be a full one! This substance certainly offered us a rich, full, extremely rewarding day.

## *2C-T-8*

Every once in a while a new compound comes down the pike which is particularly outstanding, the greatly sought-after elixir that produces the +4 experience (see Appendix II for rating scale definitions). One never knows whether it is the special properties of the compound, the psychic state and disposition of the subject, a fortunate combination of environment and companions, a particular combination of individual body chemistry and the compound, or some composite of the above. But on the occasion of my one and only trial with 2C-T-8, all of the necessary factors were present for a memorable, outstanding experience.

2C-T-8, code name for 2,5-dimethoxy-4-cyclopropylmethylthiophenethylamine[6], is a long-acting phenethylamine compound less potent than 2C-T-2 or 2C-T-7. Here is a report of our first experience:

Jean takes 39 m.g. of 2C-T-8, I take 40 m.g. While waiting for developments, I decide to work on the novel I have been writing. For several days I have been blocked, and not able to produce anything. I become aware of many facets of the characters and the possibilities that could open up in their lives. Also, of many twists and turns the plot can take. I have enough material to keep me writing for days!

The day continues remarkably. I feel exceptionally good, there is no trace of "below the line", the customary sludginess I always have to work through, and I achieve a state of monumental insight and understanding. This is a real awakening, as though I had never before known how to properly use these compounds.

I see myself as a fantastic computer. I am infinite being, with all resources contained in my vastness. Anything I wish to see is like pressing the keys on a computer keyboard to call up a particular file. In this case, the key is the focus of my attention. As I hold a central thought in my mind it unfolds, revealing the contents of the file. I have an absolutely marvelous time for several hours operating my computer, examining various concepts. Some of the key words I focus on are:

a. Love. As I look at Jean to feel my love for her, I realize that loving is not just seeing God at the core of the person – God is part of the whole being, including the ego and all the person's idiosyncrasies. As Jean moves around, I delight in watching every little movement. As I direct love at myself, I encounter a lot of resistance. I keep holding love, and come to peace with much of myself. At one point I get a glimpse of my soul, or Anima – that fantastically beautiful Feminine Presence that is a figure of radiance and light which fills everything with wonder.

I find the title of Jampolsky's book *Love is Letting Go of Fear* an excellent guide. By replacing with love the initial fear I often feel when I release to explore inside, the fear dissipates and indeed turns to love. This is also a good way to deal with anger.

b. Peace. A most wondrous thing to feel out and experience.

c. Gratitude. Gratitude is certainly a major key to life. When observing with gratitude, it affirms the beauty and reality of the focus of attention. This in turn reveals more depth to be grateful for. Which increases gratitude. This rises to incredible heights of experience, and floods through all aspects of life. Marvelous, marvelous. Being grateful for Jean, I discover that she is a perfect partner for me.

d. Jean. Jean has gone through a struggle of whether she wanted to live or die. She is terribly afraid of being alone. We are able to talk very openly and honestly. We are extremely grateful to be with each other, and to share this experience just with the two of us. We acknowledge our need for each other. She is doing very honest work, going deeply and comprehensively into her feelings.

As we discuss loneliness, we confirm that once we discover our true inner being we are never alone. Yet there is great joy and wonder in being with and sharing energy with others. We realize that we do a lot to shut each other out. This ultimately builds a wall within us which shuts us off from life. We agree to stay open to each other.

When Jean goes to the studio to paint, I find loneliness creep in. I define myself as confident, able, and enjoying my work. I soon feel a wonderful sense of freedom. I release my dependence on having other people around. I now enjoy being at my computer while Jean is in the studio painting.

e. Prostate. As I examine my prostate difficulty, I see my problem is not properly handling waste. This is symbolized by not being able to empty my bladder. I pick up a lot of psychic garbage in life, as well as physical junk I have a hard time throwing away. I resolve to dispose of waste. [Several years later, while I have made quite a bit of progress, I still need to be much tougher on this score!]

f. Anger. In my meditation the following morning, I am surprised to run into monumental anger. I find this stems from being deprived of intimacy. I generate even more anger by trying to convince myself that I don't really need intimacy and can exist self-sufficiently. I feel a great deal of benefit from discharging this anger and replacing it with love. It seems clear that holding back anger could well be responsible for the swelling of the prostate gland. An interesting item to research.

This has been a most productive experience, and at the same time was free of discomfort. Therefore we were surprised to hear that with other experimenters there were as many negatives as positives. 2C-T-8 consequently has not been actively pursued. I am left with the dilemma of how I can have such a remarkable experience on a substance that many others find unsatisfactory!

### Chapter 5 Notes

1. Shulgin, A. T. & Shulgin, A. *PIHKAL, A Chemical Love Story*. Berkeley, California: Transform Press, 1991, pp. 764-8.
2. Ibid., pp. 557-61.
3. Ibid., pp. 567-71.
4. Ibid., pp. 586-90.
5. Ibid., pp. 561-4.
6. Ibid., pp. 571-3.

# Chapter 6
# A Most Remarkable Material, 2C-E

In my thirty-five years of experimenting with old and new psychoactive agents, one stands out in my mind above all the others. It may be because of my particular temperament and value system. It may be because I like to find favorites and invest myself in them, whereby they then take on the holy glow of my special consideration.

Whatever the reason, I try very hard to be objective, and information on the efficacy of this particular substance has come in from many directions. Most all of the input confirms my belief in its special efficacy. My view that it focuses on our difficulties is not particularly confirmed, although most agree with the outstanding results.

The substance is 2C-E, code name for 2,5-dimethoxy-4-ethylphenethylamine[1]. Its depth of profound activity had been discovered many years prior to my use. Much of this time had been taken to assure that its power was manageable and could be truly useful to others. My first use was when I was completing recovery from surgery. I feel that it added substantially to my recovery rate, as well as having other outstanding characteristics.

For me, 2C-E turned out to be the most powerful truth serum I have ever encountered. It seemed to absolutely insist that I become completely honest and face my difficulties. As I got into the experience, I became quite uncomfortable. This was a massive, amorphous, unidentifiable discomfort that clung to me. I rapidly learned that the discomfort stemmed from the unresolved difficulties in my life. Many of these are discussed in detail in the reports that follow. As I confronted these difficulties and dealt with them, they subsided. I was then able to enter powerful, transforming experiences.

At first, tinges of uneasiness would stay with me throughout the day. I felt that the substance refused to let go of me until I resolved the problem producing the stress. This often kept with me well into the night, although there would be frequent waves of outstanding splendor.

The next day (except for the very first trial) all traces of the discomfort vanished. I would feel rejuvenated, renewed, full of new life and new vigor. These positive feelings would stay with me longer than with any other substance. It was as though something very real had changed inside, so that part of my inner being was transformed in a more complete way than with other substances.

I would most always feel that I had risen to a new level of being, and had broken through to a new kind of freedom and joy. However, much to my disappointment, this state was short-lived, and I would lapse back to previous habits where I would become subject to being tired and sometimes out of sorts. But as time went on with repeated experiences, I spent less time in the uncomfortable states and more in true enjoyment of the experience. Likewise, my day-to-day life held up better in the comfortable, enjoyable spaces. And after two years, and with somewhat lighter doses, I could spend the whole day's experience in very enjoyable states!! These euphoric states are closely correlated with the most significant kinds of learning.

Below are excerpts from some of the detailed reports of my experiences with 2C-E over a three year period:

> My first experience with 2C-E: I am at a low point in my life. I'm very weak from surgery, and I'm very depleted from the lack of exercise.
>
> I take 12 m.g. of 2C-E, selecting from the known range of 10 to 20 m.g. In the early hours I move through quite a bit of heavy stuff, but I accept it gracefully. In the middle and late afternoon I reach an enormously rewarding, exalted state.
>
> In about 40 minutes from starting, I feel slightly squeamish. I lie on the sofa, looking out the window. I feel very heavy. I accept this and enjoy the view. It feels great to lie down, relax, let go.
>
> I examine a sacramental ritual worked out by a good, knowledgeable friend. It focuses me in a rewarding direction and leaves some of the discomfort behind.
>
> I find it rewarding to sit up in a meditating position; it immediately intensifies the experience. I remember hearing a Bartholomew[2] tape yesterday saying achieving spiritual awakening is like birth, moving from a confined area to expansion. This is certainly happening to me now. Walls dissolve and I rapidly expand into space with marvelous elation. Then I begin to feel fear. I simply breath through the fears, and as I do this, they dissolve and are replaced by a comforting elation.
>
> I lie down again. I experience the enormous intoxication of power. I am very taken with it; it feels marvelous to have and exert power. Examining the attraction of power, I am struck with a deep, deep sense of failure. I feel inept and completely unsuccessful as a writer. In fact I have developed no skills at all other than intellectual. Even with the thing I feel best at, sharing sacramental journeys, Jean does most of the work and I do very little to help host our guests. I feel my unworthiness far stronger than ever before. I see the deep Jewish pattern of developing intellectual and highly critical mental faculties with no genuine warmth. In fact, it makes us very critical of others, and unliked. I also profoundly feel again that projects for solving mankind's problems are very inappropriate if we can't get along with the person we live with. I see how very primitive is the evolution of mankind; we are still in the earliest stages of development. Because of our powerful egos, it is extremely hard to get along with the one other person we live with, much less additional ones in the same household. It seems almost hopeless for groups to learn to live together. I see why two different groups that I know are trying to develop satisfactory communities. While I don't know any that really work, I become much more sympathetic to their efforts.
>
> Meditating again and holding my mind steady, a deep, extremely profound and powerful light grows within, completing revitalizing my insides. I keep meditating, but can't hold the focus. I realize that I must express gratitude for such a profound experience and balance it with activity in the world, not just keep seeking more experience.
>
> Outside I am fascinated by the loveliness of the sky and the way the clouds light up. We dwell on gratitude, which makes everything open up more and more beautifully. All shades of discomfort, tiredness, and lethargy are gone. My body feels rejuvenated, overwhelmed with beauty. There is a marvelous flow of energy and feeling between Jean and me. Clouds are incredible, and come fully

to life as I hold still to watch them. Thinking is extremely clear; there is a wonderful flow of insights.

> I decide to investigate the power of love. The beauty, love, and wonder grow indescribably as I watch. Gratitude continues to intensify it all. I feel that one need never be afraid to look and discover something, because if you don't search with love, you won't be able to find it. Our fear prevents the opening. When one searches with love, the love overcomes the fear and opens the door. If one is afraid of death, one won't find out anything significant about death until one looks with love. And it seems to me that whatever one looks for with love is discovered.

> Jean leaves and I sit on the deck to watch the clouds. I feel loneliness at her departure. I accept this and look at it, and find I can't be alone while realizing God is with me. I become absorbed in His presence, watching the beauty. I then realize that everything I am looking at is me, and as I look around at the beauty and feel gratitude, I am playing with myself! This is a fantastic feeling. I watch the dogs sitting quietly on the deck, totally attuned to the sounds they hear, the energies that surround us. They appear to have an enormous capacity to thoroughly enjoy themselves by being in tune with all of nature around them.

> Taking the dogs for a last evening walk, the loneliness comes over me again. I feel loneliness as the greatest human problem, and see we can do an enormous service to relieve the pain of others if we can help them to learn to look for their fulfillment in God, where they need never be lonely again. My own loneliness disappears as I turn my attention to resolving the loneliness of others. This seems axiomatic: my own pain disappears as I am concerned for others.

2C-E is a truly remarkable material. It is powerful, and helped me work through some extremely heavy negative feelings. With a reasonably light dose, it permits exploring the vastness and the exalted as well as anything I know, and better than most. It is a wonderful substance, and richly deserves much more exploration.

While this first introduction to 2C-E was extremely rewarding, I felt there were still areas within me requiring resolution. So two weeks later I repeated the experience with a somewhat higher dose, 15 m.g.:

> I am struck by a thought, had I ever said I wish I'd never been born??? I seem to have one time said this or thought it deeply. I look around; I can feel very little appreciation for life or for my surroundings. As I look at myself over the past, I see much unhappiness. Am I really enjoying life? I don't feel enthused about anything. Am I ready to die?

> I close my eyes to seek inwardly for an answer. I find I am extremely frightened by growing old. I am desperately trying to stay alive, trying so hard that I am using energy that would keep me alive for a long time. I fetch a mirror to examine myself. As I look, I feel I am much too involved with myself. I need to turn my attention to the welfare of others. It feels preferable to be more concerned for Jean's well-being. I must learn to overcome the inertia that keeps me from doing things.

> Apparently something within me won't forgive. I decide to once and for all look deeply into my past to see if something happened to me that is the source of all of this misery. I remember from last time to look with love. It is hard work searching with the light of love, but it is extremely rewarding. As I lovingly search it is very pleasant, and a lot of deeply repressed material re-

leases. It feels superb. Very striking, pronounced imagery begins to flow, as a beautifully-colored, flowing fluid. It is marvelous to watch; it requires holding very still.

I am feeling much better, and I take the dogs out for a walk. I am again overcome by loneliness; I simply breathe through it. I feel a great, awesome sense of trust for the universe. We have unending ingenuity to solve all problems and make life wonderful for everyone, if we can develop the correct attitude.

I think again about the problem of how very difficult it is for people to learn to get along with each other. I feel I am living my life as a test of whether this can be done. Can two people who often don't like each other learn to love and care for each other? I brought Jean out here away from everything so that we completely confront each other and learn how to do this. For all it's ups and downs, it's working!

I start up a hill, and it seems there is a light shining down from above. I postulate in my mind that when I reach the top of the hill, I will be in glory. I reach the top, and I am!! I am surrounded by light and beauty. The clouds are all lit up, revealing enormous splendor! I am overwhelmed with euphoria. At last, I thought, I have the secret to becoming creator. I need only to think and imagine remarkable things, and they will come to pass. I felt this is what happened: my mind projected it, and then a more powerful inner force brought it into reality. I am absolutely elated. I sit down to do more. But it won't work!!

I am thoroughly dismayed, and sink into depression. I didn't have the secret after all. I look at the mountains and become still. I become aware of the old Buddhist axiom of not striving. It seems clear that if I pour my energy into creating beauty and euphoria, this simultaneously creates an empty hole which I will subsequently experience as the opposite. The answer is equanimity – let things be as they are.

I remain still for a while. I am so still I can hear all the rumblings within my body – my heart beating, the blood circulating. I become so still that I can hear the very heart of creation. It lasts only a second, but enough to convince me that in that stillness is the source of everything.

Several times during the day I was able to look up into the light and draw myself into a higher, more wonderful state of being.

Jean comes home while I am just returning from outdoors. I am in a strange space, not elated nor enthused, feeling rather empty. I feel perhaps I had taken too large a dose, and had no volition over the experience. And it was more fun when Jean accompanied me. Jean puts on some peppy music, and I am transformed. I dance freely, energetically, and all vestiges of ill feeling disappear. I gather energy as I dance, and am elated. Physical movement brings an exhilarating transformation.

That evening I realize that I really am creating my life more wholesomely, that focusing on good thoughts and outcomes does bring results. I feel I have opened a whole new door to life.

We continue our explorations of 2C-E. I have two major personal goals. The first is to resolve the heavy feelings I accumulate with the passage of time. The other is to become as free as possible, and explore the farthest reaches of the mind. The obstacles to both these objectives were discussed in the latter part of Chapter 2, pages 34-36.

Another experience: Jean and I worked a lot on our communication, finding 2C-E an excellent material with which to develop honesty. A very profound insight into my relationship to Jean is realizing that the discomfort I experience with her is not the result of what Jean is doing to me, but what I am doing to her! After all, why should the intelligence that runs the universe make us suffer for what other people do? It is our own actions for which we must account. It took a great deal of honesty to permit this realization.[3]

Some important spiritual realizations came in the following experience:

I have taken 12 m.g. of 2C-E, followed by 3 m.g. more some two hours later. I lie down and release to the experience. As usual I feel fear, but I also feel trust. It is an enormous relief to just let go to developments. It is very difficult to stay tuned in to what I call the interface with God,[4] but this is the most worthwhile thing I can do. I feel release and cleansing, dissipating the tensions within me. I go through myriads of feelings, some of them incredibly intense. They include powerful anger, feelings of expansion to the exploding point, deep, deep inner tensions that wrack my body like a birth experience. Sometimes the anger is so great that I feel that it could break the very bones within my body. I would not be surprised if few persons choose to go through such discomfort. I wonder if advanced meditators have covered this ground, or if it is necessary for others. I find it best not to think about what's happening, but just stay tuned in and allow to happen what wants to happen. This brings sublime relief.

Late in the afternoon we sit on the deck. The sky is full of clouds, and is absolutely beautiful. I look out, thinking that this is all me. I remember both Richard Moss[5] and Bartholomew saying that we are already whole. I begin to experience this.

I get into the mode of prayer. I thought I had recently mastered this in my everyday life, but it dissipated away. Now it is in full force. I very much feel God's presence. I look Him in the face (as nearly as I can project Him directly in front of me!) and ask Him to show me myself. He immediately does so. I find it extremely difficult to sit still enough to receive the answer, but I do it. As I relax and let go, I see the incredible beauty of the sky and my surroundings, and understand that this is me. Tensions build up in my body, and I know this is resisting. So I relax more and let God reach in and heal. He is so very, very gentle, if I just let go and allow His penetration. A brilliant light grows in the clouds, with enormous power, beauty, and light. It feels very satisfying to have it happen spontaneously, rather than my making it happen.

Then I grow empty; the exalted feeling is gone. I simply relax and let it happen. Then I find myself looking at the cold, heartless core of myself that I first experienced in a previous experience with my son. I observe it for a while, and then a powerful anger grows in me. I realize that I am the Anti-Christ!! Everywhere, I move to defeat God and His goodness. I try to seduce God by being kind and loving, to use His ways, but actually I want to destroy Him and all His works![6]

Then a marvelous thing happens. As I sit looking at my rebelliousness, a subtle feeling begins to grow in my gut. It grows stronger and stronger. Then I realize it is God's love! It continues to grow stronger, and I discover that He loves me despite whatever I do, no matter how much I am against Him. This is an utterly indescribable love, binding all of creation. It is truly unconditional love, the most perfect model we can emulate.

The clouds have become incredibly beautiful. It is impossible to find the words to describe them. They are alive and charged with meaning. My perception of them is crystal clear, and it is profoundly moving to watch them. With the sharpness of every minute detail, varying shades of light and color, moving patterns and shapes, they exemplify the indescribable nature of pure being.

This is one of the greatest experiences of my life, surpassed only by the one in 1963 when I became God. But I feel that today's realization is more profound and will be more accessible, since so much has been cleared away in order for me to feel it. It is glorious to bask in, to be this love. I realize that it is there all the time, and it is simply a case of letting it in, becoming it.

After a while I begin to feel empty again. I realize that I did not express appreciation for the outstanding grace I experienced, and instead am looking to intensify it. I spend some time in gratitude and appreciation, which restores elation, bringing back all the good feelings in full intensity.

2C-E is remarkable, the most effective psychedelic of which I know. It attacks the inner dross, and while it is not always pleasant, it is tremendously rewarding, bringing great honesty and clarity. I look forward to additional exploration.

Ten days later: I have had better retention of this experience than any previous one. I am still plagued with the problem of backsliding, but I'm handling it better.

. . . . . . .

In the following experience, some very interesting phenomena occurs:

Our friend Gil is with us. I have taken 12 m.g. of 2C-E. Gil and Jean have opted for another substance. He feels he has a lot of important work to do.

Gil is stewing in his problems. I am feeling very heavy, and decide to take a supplement. Gil tells me I don't need it. I know he is right, remembering the last time we were together that things cleared up when we faced and resolved issues. I feel we need to do the same here. It works!

Later we are outside drinking in our surroundings. Again I am feeling bogged down. I decide to look inside as I try the same approach of allowing myself to feel the feelings in hopes of resolving them. But this time it comes to me that this is an old habit, and I now have lots of evidence that it takes a new direction of focus. I look up into the sky, which is filled with beautiful clouds. I begin to get an amazing sense of energy there, and I open myself to allow it to flow in. It does, and everything starts to change. I allow love to come in and wash away the old feelings. The beauty of the clouds grows to incredible intensity, and the feeling of love among us grows in proportion.

It is an outstanding day, with a superbly beautiful assortment of clouds. There is a giant, long lenticular cloud, starting about 15 miles to the north and extending southward, covering us and beyond to the south. The lenticular cloud has many layers of rounded, smooth surfaces, built on one another. In addition, there are spaces in the clouds revealing many different layers of formations, and these are moving in different directions. As we look up we are overcome by the remarkable feeling of aliveness, the continual movement, the vastness and spaciousness. We observe the delicacy of design in different clouds, varying from mists to ripples to eddies to strings of cotton and lace. All are in a vast, alive, moving whole, radiating enormous energy. We are completely captivated. And behind it all is an enormous sense of Presence.

Gil and I both feel the infinite energy source that is radiating into and filling the sky. I express how powerful is the mind of man, that we can shut all of this down until we are oblivious to it. I pray to be as open as possible, and accept it as fully as I can.

I practice being very still, which allows things to open further and become more profound. I experiment with holding the thought of love, which allows copious volumes of love to mobilize and pour into us, the surroundings, and the world. I verbalize what I am feeling, "When two or more are gathered in my name, there will I be also". Jean asked, "Why two?" I have had a lot of experience lately in feeling the Presence while alone, but the presence of the others definitely deepens considerably the feeling and profoundness of the love I am experiencing.

I can't imagine what could be more beautiful or more blissful than what we are experiencing together. Earlier in the day I had had trouble feeling deep closeness to both Jean and Gil. Now the closeness and communion are overpowering. I delight in looking up at the clouds and playing with my mind. Is it best to simply hold still, or to choose an issue for my mind to focus on and let the universe unfold it? It works both ways, and seems best to switch back and forth, as if sticking to one dynamic gets overdone. At times I feel tension rising in my body, as I am so invested in pouring out love. I realize I don't need to do this, and relax, allowing the love to flow in from the Source.

Now a new phenomena commences. As the sun descends behind the mountain, the sky fills with amazing colors – wonderful purples, pinks, even some green, and delicate shades of blue where there are no clouds. It is incredible, nothing like anything ever seen in my life; some of the colors I have never seen before. We walk around the house to see various parts of the sky, as the display is going on everywhere. Each direction yields a different pattern.

Then we notice something that we can't believe or account for. The sun is now set comfortably behind the western mountains, but in the east, rays of light are shining forth as from a new sunrise! We watch for quite a while, and the rays change somewhat and get more intense. But we can't unravel what is causing it. It seems to us to have very special significance, such as a new dawn for mankind.

This show goes on for at least three hours. Another strange thing happens. As the sun sets, the huge lenticular cloud hanging over the valley and suspended over our heads grows dark. But then it lights up again, with a wonderful cream color! This lasts another half hour, and is as inexplicable as the rays in the east.

We are all very grateful and very moved by this display. It seems to have special significance tied in with our experience. Especially as the huge, lenticular cloud dissipates and shrinks, the body of it stays directly over us.

We are deeply impressed with the enormous power that has appeared from beyond the range of our ordinary perceptions. We are filled with awe at the unfathomed mystery of creation, and this direct demonstration of how little we ordinarily apprehend. Gratitude fills us to overflowing, and we re-dedicate our search to the unfolding of the Mystery.

. . . . . . .

## Still further exploration with 15 m.g. of 2C-E:

In summary, this is an extremely intense experience, with agonizing wrenching away of deeply buried, highly impacted core debris, permitting me to rise to a profound level of realization and understanding beyond previous experience. I reach a state of great clarity. I understand with considerable depth my preoccupation with miserable feelings, and how to deal with them. Also, the painful but near complete scourging away of resistance and repressed material opens the door to a more continuing state of well-being.

At two hours the experience is wild, I am extremely energized, almost jittery, but I can't get into a space of feeling good. None of the impressive things I felt in the last experience, like God's unconditional love, seem available. I have a brief period of doubt wondering if I should have taken so much so soon after my last trial without spending more time integrating. Then I remember my goals and close my eyes and go to work.

For the next couple of hours I release to inner experience, staying focused on my feelings and working through them. I go through myriads of intense feeling – deep anger, powerful tensions – much more intense and deeper than the previous experience. I feel I am cleaning up debris down deeply in my core, and feel very good about what I am doing. As I work through these deep feelings, I feel better and gain more volition. This goes on for several hours.

I look at different situations and see with remarkable clarity. I look over my recent visit to Texas and clearly see my dynamics with several individuals that left unresolved feelings. Through forgiveness I am able to feel genuine love for the parties concerned.

All this time I am surrendering to the experience, using what volition I have to simply stay focused on what is happening. Then it occurs to me that I must take a more active role. I feel I must grab the torch and carry the light of love into the dark places, clear up the agony and suffering. This is very hard work, since I feel so tired and the resistance is so great. But with determination I get it started, and then God moves in and helps me. It begins to work beautifully, and my whole experience turns around. This becomes an incredible endeavor. I see that this is my role, to be a channel for God to carry His light into the dark places. I am overcome with emotion and the magnificent feeling of God's Presence and appreciation. Mere words cannot possibly describe the beauty, satisfaction, and fulfillment of this understanding.

After feeling exalted, I lapse back into uncomfortable feelings. But I realize that my job is to move in and clean these up with love. Instead of looking at the feeling, trying to understand it, living through it, I recognize the negative feeling as an indicator to where love needs to move in. I focus love on the negative feeling, and see that this is my role, – to relieve whatever agony and pain I can see anywhere by being a channel for bringing in the light of love. It is the highest service, and requires a willingness to face deep pain, which I had certainly done a good part of the day. This isn't easy, and I can see clearly why I have avoided it. However, the knowledge of God's power and love makes one a willing instrument, whatever the cost. I feel very rewarded and privileged.

Jean has gone to her favorite chair by her desk, and I go to sit with her and watch her. I go through my feelings of being inadequate as a man, and feel energy swell within me. I turn on some dynamic music and we dance. Energy surges through me, and I am overcome with realization after realization of love. I feel God pouring through me, and that I am an open channel. The feelings are indescribable. I am inordinately privileged and full of joy, for as I dance, God is dancing, and He appreciates me making it possible for Him to do so. And everything around me, like our cat, relishes this opportunity to be with God. I easily assume different roles and postures. I am a wild young lover, and

> quickly change to a creaking old man, which I delightfully demonstrate by hobbling bent over around the room.
>
> Then I am a ballet dancer, followed by a curious child. I am full of fun and joy, and at the same time enormously overcome by the sheer wonder, beauty, and ecstasy of it all. Then I feel very blessed for having made and stuck to my commitment to Jean. Many times it has been tough and very uncomfortable, but now I am reaping the rewards. I would never have rooted out these deep barriers in my soul unless I had relentlessly pursued seeking love in this relationship.

This experience turned out to be one of the very principal, formative experiences of all of my explorations into the Greater Self. It had an enormous impact, and was of outstanding significance. Here I was presented with what seemed to me to be the most exalted role that man can perform, to be a full-fledged, totally responsible partner of the Divine, totally committed to carrying out the highest purposes of the Divine. While I was far from being in the position to fulfill such a mission, the requirements of it were presented in crystal clarity.

First, I felt that no one is asked to undertake such a mission. It is arrived at through gratitude for the wonder and magnificence of creation, and the desire to give back some small measure of the prodigious bounties one has received. I am sure that there is gratitude throughout the cosmos for each individual who willingly subscribes to this assignment.

Second, the full implications seem extremely difficult to realize. For it seems to me that one cannot perceive the full range of possibilities without first clearing out one's own personal limitations. This is an extremely difficult, and for me very painful thing to do. The difficulties are enormously compounded when one realizes that they are not one's own personal difficulties that must be faced and resolved. For heightened awareness reveals that I am one with all of creation. As I discovered in my very first psychedelic experience, I am one, part and parcel with all of humanity. And as I realize this, and appreciate the enormity of the gifts of all of humanity in which I share, I simultaneously realize that I share the pain and suffering of all of humanity. So it is not only my own personal shadow I must confront and resolve, but the collective shadow of all mankind!

I can not help but wonder why it is necessary to go through all of this pain and suffering. But one thing was very deeply impressed upon me. The more willing I became to confront this vast array of agony, the more aware I became of the unfathomed, unending supply of love that was available to counter it. And it was not up to me personally to vanquish the misery and suffering of mankind. This can only be done by the redeeming love of God. And because of the dictum of Free Will, God's love can best be brought into play by willing participants who consciously agree to be channels for this love. This means being willing to stand before the most horrible and agonizing conditions and focus the energy of love upon them. The redeeming power is in the love itself, and comes directly from the Supreme Source. Yet regardless of the willingness of those who play this role and the power of the universal force that supports them, what is actually received depends on the openness and willingness of the recipient.

I doubt if one enters into such realization suddenly. For myself, it was the growing awareness of God's love and light that increased my trust and encouraged the willingness to go deeper into my pain, which also made the pain continually less uncomfortable.

Many of these conditions are outlined in Joseph Campbell's outstanding book *The Hero with A Thousand Faces*. Here the journey is presented as viewed in a great variety of cultures. The basic elements of the journey are the same: the call and search, undergoing trials, the discovery of the redeeming Father, and the return to the world to aid in the redemptive process. "The problem of the hero going to meet the father is to open his soul beyond terror to such a degree that he will be ripe to understand how the sickening and insane tragedies of this vast and ruthless cosmos are completely validated in the majesty of Being."[7]

. . . . . . .

This is the first of a series of planned investigations to explore different dose ranges with 2C-E:

> I take 12 m.g. 2C-E. I have my typical initial period, working through a lot of heavy material by lying still and confronting it. We have recently returned from a ten day tour of Hawaii with Bartholomew, where much of the instruction was on deepening our meditation. While I learned a lot and benefited significantly, it is immediately apparent to me that the efficacy of meditation for realizing a clear state of being can not at all compare to the use of these substances. I really need this experience to improve my state of well-being.
>
> Wondering why I am so tired, I discover deep anger at growing old. I terribly resent it and the bodily discomforts that accompany it – stiffness, arthritic symptoms, stiff neck, less energy. I resent the loss of my powers. I see I need to grow old gracefully. My fussing over it only makes it worse.
>
> I walk outside to my flat rock (see description of the flat rock in Appendix III, Procedure). I am besieged with a variety of points of view. I see my struggle for goodness and light, the conflicting horrors of the world, the different positions of others. It all seems like nonsense. Then an overwhelming insight descends on me: The whole purpose of life is simply to enjoy!! If it's no fun, forget it.
>
> Listening to the Berlioz Requiem, I am flooded with admiration for Berlioz's skill as a composer and the sheer magnitude and beauty of the composition, as well as the skill of the performers. I am immediately moved to a profound level of love. It seems the most beautiful composition I have ever heard, astounding in content, creativeness, and performance. At one point, I see death like a troop of Hitler's Gestapo, marching toward me. It is intermingled with the light produced by the beautiful soprano voices. Death is not threatening.
>
> Then the horn crescendo bursts forth with the most incredible honor to God imaginable. I ride with it, but I am not completely immersed in the music. Part of me is holding back, mocking. I feel my total independence, total reluctance to being told what to do, my colossal arrogance. Then another utterly outstanding passage sweeps me completely away. No matter what I do – rape, murder, cheat, lie, steal – God still loves me!! I am totally undone, and cannot contain my sobbing. The profundity and absolute constancy of God's love is be-

yond comprehension. Jean is having a full blown experience just being present. I pray to learn to love with the kind of love I have just experienced.

This was incredibly moving, and released all the inner tension and unresolved feelings I had been experiencing. We hear the rest of the music in phenomenal joy and delight.

The rest of the day goes beautifully. I am in a wonderful space of clarity, and can examine many different things. Sitting on the deck with Jean, I become aware of many aspects of her beauty. A marvelous feeling of peace steals over us. The world around us is filled with beauty and the Presence of the One. If a discomfort arises, I focus God on it, and it resolves. However, I find that if I try to make this a rule, it stops working. It is only by maintaining a live, deep interconnection with God that He joins me in my endeavors. Otherwise it is the ego taking over to establish its own power. But in general, discomfort and negative experiences are melted in love.

I think about the differences between 2C-E and LSD. As great as the latter is, with its outstanding clarity and beauty, this somehow feels more kindly, more strongly centering, more fruitful. Who knows whether this is a genuine difference in substances, or a reflection of the work that has been done, or some other factor? What I can say is that it is an amazing working material, with a very great deal getting accomplished.

During the day, I become aware of my enormous self-hatred. Also, I clearly see that the things I resent in Jean's behavior are simply a reflection of my own poor behavior. At one point, sitting on the deck with Jean and pondering different relationships, it seems clear that no matter who you chose as a partner, you will probably end up reflecting to each other the other's worst characteristics, calling for resolution. I again see my own reluctance to put myself out much for others, and this results in a very uncomfortable energy block within me.

I think over the day's experience. What a marvelous, outstanding day!! I encountered a great deal of my own unnecessary baggage, and 2C-E, as I claim, seems to burn it up. And as the dross burns away, the light can come through. I am enormously grateful, especially the next day, when I feel completely rejuvenated and whole. I am very glad I stuck with the low dose. The feelings encountered were at times quite uncomfortable, but I realize that they are me, and that it's very important to be at home with them. Clearing them up, or being willing to ride through them, permits an outstanding high level experience for me.

Watching the sundown while walking out on the rocks is a marvelous experience. I am completely at peace all alone, an important achievement for me. It seems clear that the very best I can do, both for me and the state of the world, is to simply be fully who I am. If I can maintain this state, it will automatically work out the best for everyone.

As the underlying negative feelings dissipate, I am left with a wonderful sense of well-being that perceives everything that happened in an exalted light. I very much appreciate the uniqueness of my own being, and see that we each have our own experience to offer. I can be proud to contribute what I experience without trying to prove anything or convince anyone.

A good uphill climb following this experience proved that my body was much rejuvenated. Exercise is a marvelous way to integrate the experience and throw off some of the residue left after a hard working day. I found I had dropped my concerns about aging, and many of the bodily symptoms of aging were gone.

. . . . . . .

I set up this day to take a light dose of 2C-E. It is my hope that the lighter amount will elevate me into higher energy than normal, allow me to accomplish the ordinary tasks of the day more efficiently, and enjoy a higher state of "Presence". I also hope to learn to overcome resistances to chores, as has happened with previous small doses of other substances. In addition, I wish to find out if the dose will be light enough to not stir up the deep, uncomfortable feelings I almost always encounter with this substance.

I take 8 m.g. of 2C-E. I decide to work on a paper I had once started on how this material level of creation came into being. I think the paper starts well, but I can't see how to continue past where I had stopped before, when single-celled life came into being.

I lie on the sofa. I realize I don't know shit. How preposterous, to speculate creation!! I don't even know how an amoeba came into being, or if anyone does!

I look at the vastness of the unknown. I can see how fearless exploration with these substances might lead to gaining knowledge of how life came into being. I realize that the universe has been created in love. Then I experience the roaring anger of not knowing, which brings me back to the keyboard to write again. The following are my live notes:

> This is a raging, raging anger. I don't know, and I absolutely hate not knowing, but at the same time I don't want to do what it takes to learn!! What a dilemma!! The dilemma of the world!!
>
> At two hours, this is getting very intense. I am surprised at the intensity. I am typing perfectly!!! This is a real change, as I ordinarily fill the page with typos. I am going through a great struggle. I feel the need to stay conscious, in control, master inner feelings and work as a conscious human being. Right now this feels good ...
>
> Ten hours later: I had decided to go to my meditation rock (described in Appendix III). When I arrived there, I was feeling awful, dragging a heavy load. I was out of breath and had to force myself to climb the hill, which I was determined to do. A brief look around did not bring my accustomed contact with the Numinous. I lay back and relaxed with eyes closed.
>
> I would really be a writer if I could describe what happened. I simply put myself in the hands of God, and all the discomfort began to slide away. This contact is the only contact in life that is important. It leads to everything worthwhile. But mostly it permits simply settling into what we really are, our true inner Self. Here I am tempted to use flowery adjectives, or expansive descriptions. But no, it is simply who we are. Resting there, being there, is beyond any description. Wonder? Glory? Profundity? As far as I can stretch my mind, the adjectives won't do. All the little devices, the little tricks I used to use to encourage me into this state, all seem terribly inept and even manipulative. Allowing? Letting? Are these better words? As I struggle for expression, the feeling once again comes over me. I want to do everything I possibly can to encourage it, to deepen it, to remember it in a way that can never be forgotten. All I can do is ask. The rest is up to Him.
>
> But that's not true. I can do a lot! Prepare the way for the Lord! I see myself shouting, screaming, calling forth glorious music. Yes, prepare a way! And that way is an emptying out, a total cleansing so that He may enter an untarnished room, free of any dross whatsoever, and fill it with His radiance. Don't put new wine in old wineskins. But

> how can we possibly make it clean enough, pure enough for His Holiness?
>
> Only in the clean, pure fire of love. Nothing else will do. It is love that burns out the dross. It is love that purifies and cleanses.
>
> Light the fire of 2C-E! Let the flames burn away the dross, burnish the core of radiance that awaits to shine forth!

I was stuck with this concept of creating the clean space, what it really means, and is it truly necessary? Not knowing how to proceed, I abandoned my writing. Now, three days later, being driven through the Owens Valley of Eastern California, I am continuing my report:

> It is strange that just rereading what I wrote before and starting to think about it considerably raises my consciousness as I look at the mountains around me. This drive through the Owens Valley is a truly outstanding one. Surrounded by towering mountains on both sides of the valley, the views are very inspiring. I was blocked at the time by what it meant to prepare the clear space. Now as I think about it, it is what I have been saying for some time. The cleanliness is the purity of mind, the creating of the clear, empty space that God can enter. We don't throw away our past experiences or our memories, but it is our consciousness that we clear.
>
> It is interesting that we spent the day yesterday hiking in the mountains with a student of Tibetan Buddhist meditation. We discussed a number of factors concerning reaching and maintaining a stable, clear mind. I have to say at this point in time that the best aid I know to getting the most realization from these psychedelic experiences, as well as on a day-to-day basis, is the mind training of utter stillness. It is this stillness which allows the Celestial to manifest itself in our consciousness, and to become our constant companion.

This trial with only 8 m.g. of 2C-E brought forth many lessons. The outstanding ones are:

1. To set intention with full consciousness.

2. Having set intention, to not let feelings interfere. The fact that I am uncomfortable is no reason not to carry out the intention. I feel I have grown a lot in inner strength today by my willingness to act despite how I felt. Of course if the feelings are powerful, I must sit down and resolve them. Two good ways: The best is to surrender completely to the Divine, or Inner Teacher, and allow developments and understanding to unfold. This usually dissolves the feelings and often brings understanding. Another very useful technique is Gendlin's focusing procedure,[8] which helps to rapidly arrive at the core of the feelings and obtain release. But there is something also to be said for simply growing in inner strength sufficiently to ignore some of the habitual responses and drop them by the wayside.

3. Willingness to act. I am recognizing more frequently a deep slothfulness within me. It might be based in anger; a large component is no doubt the sheer habit of laziness developed in childhood, when I was well taken care of by solicitous parents and didn't have to put myself out. Taking action focuses and generates energy and overcomes resistance.

4. Energy is mobilized by the depth of intention. This experience gave me an excellent opportunity to experience my resistances, and deepening intention mobilized the strength to dissolve them away. It has consequently left me with more energy and freedom of action.

5. Learning to relax and be in tune with my center. I became acutely aware of my compulsiveness, my anxiety to push rapidly through things, even my strained breathing. I can relax and let the universe join me in what I am doing, feel the marvelous sense of Presence, be aware of it, enjoy it, and take as much time as is necessary to get the job done. I became aware of how the mind skips over things, anticipates the end without allowing full participation in the deed. Full participation, which also means full awareness, is easy, effortless, enjoyable, competent. It is like being constantly accompanied by one's lover. This is the way I always want to function.

In summary, despite the initial discomfort, I had a most rewarding experience of Pure Being, immersed in the fullness of the One, and an impressive glimpse of the superb beauty of the feminine nature which seems to be my soul. Several hours were devoted to wearing away my internal resistances and learning to function with my feelings as they are. This resulted in a marvelous day following the experience, when I was rejuvenated, whole, full of energy, and feeling enormously competent. A hike two days after the experience was most refreshing to the body. It was my highest climb in many months, and was negotiated almost effortlessly.

I am finding that my pattern after 2C-E runs something like this: The day after is one of great rejuvenation, centeredness, strength, and energy. This is followed by some disruptions as I learn to accommodate the new energy that has been released. There may also be some fresh upheavals of new unconscious material which may take a day or two or three to integrate. Then a new steady-state condition arrives, which most of the time is on a new plateau of functioning.

With the smaller dose, this aftermath has transpired rapidly. I am awed at the power and effectiveness of such a low dose. In fact, it seems that the lower amount is much more effective in dealing with problems close to where you live, and improving day-to-day functioning.

. . . . . . .

After some absence of experiments, I am ready to focus on new exploring rather than "cleaning up" stuff. I take 12 m.g. 2C-E. Jean takes 10 m.g. Despite this resolve, I find it necessary to spend some time in the "cleaning up" process. Once through this stage, we encounter some interesting, fresh revelations:

> I lie down and close my eyes and am gripped by fear. I trust and breathe through it, finding myself flying through space. It is most gratifying to open myself to higher dimensions, from whence the rejuvenating, healing sustenance comes. Despite whatever fear or stressful feelings arise, keeping focused and letting go to this expanding edge brings a marvelous transformation of being.

I am feeling much better, and I make a comparison in my mind between 2C-E and LSD. The latter is the king of all openers, presenting the broadest, freest range of experience that I know. Yet now it seems to me that it is largely mental. The mind moves freely through all kinds of universes, but these universes can rapidly dissolve away after the experience. And I find myself involved in almost compulsive ongoing mental processes after such experiences.

2C-E, on the other hand, seems to strike much deeper within at an affective level. The changes made are much more permanent, or so it seems to me. Internal resistances, repressed feelings, and the debris that accumulates from contact with life burn off, leaving one free and whole and more strongly centered. It still requires focused attention to get the most from the experience.

I am suddenly aware of the deep, deep anguish inside of me crying for God. I see that all the pain of the world is this separation from God; this anguish is widespread. This pain is so intense that we bury it deeply, hoping never to feel it. To help us hide it, we pretend other things are important: status, accomplishments, possessions, amusements, power. But while we may temporarily enjoy such stratagem, the anguish remains undiminished until we finally address it. It may take lifetimes, but it is the only course to ultimate peace.

Then I see that I can pour in my love to help dissolve this pain. At first this feels absolutely wonderful. Then I begin to wonder, how far does this go? I don't need to support everyone, because doesn't each individual need to learn how to do this for himself?

Then an overwhelming realization descends upon me. This wondering is an intellectual attempt at escape. Even though it is true that each must resolve his/her own relationship to God, nevertheless I must give this loving support to every living being! And I can do this, because I am God, and can draw on infinite resources to support every creature! And there is no living thing that can be left out from this consideration! This is an overpowering realization. [I later discovered that it is a principle foundation of Buddhist philosophy that enlightment can be achieved only by committing oneself to the happiness and well-being of all sentient beings.]

I realize that from this point of view, the greatest service is to answer needs. The needs of every living creature everywhere demand attention, and answering them is what counts most. I can see how blind the world is to this proposition, especially with the War on Drugs and other wars, where people attempt to free themselves of their real responsibility by disposing of the offending creatures, or pursuing their own private interests.

As I sit overwhelmed with this responsibility, it comes to me that my first concern is my own partner and my own home. It is very clear that much needs to be done right here to be a demonstration of Divinity. With further reflection, I see that I don't need to go out looking for persons to help, but only need to deal with what naturally comes up for me in my life. It is also clear that looking for a way to help others can be a way of dodging one's own personal responsibility.

At five hours into the experience, I decide to see what it's like to write under the influence:

> I am beginning to feel very good. The clouds outside have an indescribable, ephemeral beauty. I could easily spend the rest of the day just watching them.
>
> But Jean says, if she were a painter, she should be in her studio painting. And if I'm a writer, I should be sitting here writing. So here I am!!

Do I want to try to recount where I've been? I don't think so. It's been tremendous, much learning, much insight. But is there some deeper, underlying principle? I can feel something deep within my breast. It is crying for expression. If I only knew how!!! Somehow it is the thing that makes everything make sense – all the ups and downs, the euphoria, the deep depression, the agony, the screaming for recognition – something underlies it all. Is it weeping? I feel that it must be, because it cares so very deeply. Now I feel helpless, because no words could ever approach it. And yet, it must take some more tangible form, some more tangible shape. I am on the edge of some great promise of what is to be. What is it??? WHAT IS IT????!!!!

A whisper of an eternal wind. What an eloquent, sublime feeling! I am annoyed because my manual skills are not paying due respect to the sublimity of experience. What is this whisper in the wind, what is this remarkable feminine Presence? I want to leave the keyboard and just experience, yet something holds me here. Oh, if I could only just let it flow through me in its utter elegance!! What would it be like to be tuned to the very center, to the fountain of utterances! And to have those utterances sublimely directed!! What word could possibly be given to account for it all?

Only one word. GRATITUDE. --------------- Gratitude. Gratitude.

Gratitude has its limits. You can only be grateful for the reality that you can perceive. Therefore to be fully grateful, one must encompass more and more reality. As I look up into the sky, I see the beauty and wonder expand enormously, and my gratitude swells with it.

What happens if one opens one's mind to what is beyond that and then beyond that and then beyond that????

I look up at the sky and expand indefinitely. Nothing specific comes. Just unending visual clarity. I hope for some accompanying feeling of bliss, like Dr. Wolff's experience I had recently read,[9] but affect was absent. Then all of a sudden, a great realization strikes me. Many people that are now being born are the ones that were pushed aside in the past by those asserting their own programs. So when you murder them and put them out of the way, they only come back!! Sooner or later we are going to have to learn to deal with them!! There's no escaping them!!! At last an answer to the theme that has been reoccurring through the last several journeys – why does the population keep exploding?

We have no choice. We must learn to get along with each other.

. . . . . . .

*Low Doses*. One of the interesting developments in the 2C-E research was the discovery of the efficacy of this substance at relatively low dose levels. Reports came in of excellent results with difficult psychiatric cases at the 10 m.g. level. Jean and I began experimenting more at this level, and found it very effective.

We found that 10 m.g. was a very appropriate introductory level for subjects with prior experience with psychedelics. In our first trials with new persons, I often warned them that my own experience with 2C-E indicated that it was a hard working material. This meant that much of the time one might be forced to confront uncomfortable feelings, so that the journey might not be pleasant. This was compensated for by the improved state of being which followed the experience.

This turned out to be inaccurate information. While it held true for me, it didn't seem to hold true for others. With at least a dozen other subjects, the experience was found not only rewarding but enjoyable. In fact, all of our trials with other persons employing 2C-E have been very fulfilling experiences, including new learning, increased bonding of participants, wonderful feelings of closeness and heightened energy, access to high level realizations, and rejuvenation following the experience.

In one case a couple who invariably had extremely uncomfortable experiences with 2C-B and 2C-T-2 found 2C-E at the 10 m.g. level very enjoyable as well as useful.

I was often surprised at the power of such a low dose. The composition of the group has a significant bearing on the ensuing results. One experience with 17 m.g. did not reach as much intensity or clarity or deep, solid, good feeling as another with 10 m.g. in a different grouping.

The section entitled Bill and Joanna in Chapter 11 contains a description of how outstanding an experience of 10 m.g. of 2C-E can be with very close friends.

. . . . . . .

In the act of recounting these experiences, I have been moved again and again by the wonder of the vistas that have been opened, the exposure of the utter goodness that underlies the universe, the inconceivable love that permeates all of creation, the incredible wonder that is Man, and the opportunities that lie before us. I am immensely grateful for having been privileged to undergo such experiences.

As I ponder the blessings that have come my way, I fervently hope that others with similar aspirations may have access to the same opportunities. May we find the determination to brave the government regulations governing research and find ways, either through taking the complex steps to compliance or through more favorable regulations, to proceed with research of these very valuable substances.

### Chapter 6 Notes

1. Shulgin, A. T. & Shulgin, A. *PIHKAL, a Chemical Love Story*. Berkeley, California: Transform Press, 1991, pp. 515-518.
2. Bartholomew is the name of an entity channeled by a very dear friend of ours, Mary-Margaret Moore. I have heard a great many tapes, and Jean and I have participated in a number of workshops and three tours guided by the Bartholomew

wisdom. I personally feel that Bartholomew is one of the greatest sources of spiritual wisdom on the planet, speaking not only to the issues of God-realization but taking into account the place where most of us live in daily functioning. I find almost all of my personal experiences in meditation and the use of the sacraments confirmed by the Bartholomew wisdom.

3. People who are innocent victims of the attack of aggressors are obvious exceptions to this concept. Yet there are those who would claim that karma may be responsible. I am not perceptive enough to observe such law of karma in action, although I have a healthy regard of it in terms of how we are subject to our inappropriate actions. I can claim with confidence that regardless of how clever we are at explaining things, what we know is a scratch on the surface of the vast Cloud of Unknowing that is contained in the Mystery. I have little doubt that our personal responsibility extends with our growth of awareness. This fact alone may deter many from seeking growth.
4. Interface with God. I have been blessed for a number of years with being aware that there is a very special place to focus my consciousness. It is like scanning the radio spectrum with a receiver, and finding the place to "tune in". At first it was very faint, but a definite place. I always found it fruitful to hold my attention there, as this is what made available perceptions and realizations beyond my usual frame of reference. In time this grew to a place of calm and then euphoria, and a more and more powerful feeling that I was in the very Presence of God. Now I treasure it as a priceless connection where the most significant realizations of my life take place. It requires a steady, quiet focus, and works best with an ability to empty the mind, cease conceptual thought, and be perfectly open to whatever happens.
5. Richard Moss is a gifted teacher who for several years maintained a conference center in the town of Lone Pine, California. He is an expert at providing situations that result in transforming experiences. See his books *The I That is We* (Millbrae, CA: Celestial Arts, 1981) and *The Black Butterfly* (Berkeley, CA: Celestial Arts, 1987).
6. It has been proposed that there are two powerful and opposite drives within us, Eros and Thanatos. Eros is considered by some to be like an archetypal drive for life, and Thanatos a corresponding drive for death. Both drives are considered to exist deeply within our psyche, and operate as natural instincts. Freud in particular proposed such a dichotomy, the life and death instincts, libido and aggression. The experience described here convinced me of the power of these drives!
7. Campbell, Joseph. *The Hero With a Thousand Faces*. Princeton, N.J.: Princeton University Press, Second Edition, 1968, p. 147.
8. Gendlin, Eugene T. *Focusing*. New York: Bantam Books, 1981. Based on extensive research, Gendlin and his associates discovered the factors important for rapid progress in therapy. See Chapter 3, note 9.
9. Merrell-Wolff, Franklin. *The Philosophy of Consciousness Without an Object*. New York: The Julian Press, Inc., 1983.

# Chapter 7
# Bummers

Most of what has been excerpted for inclusion in this volume are outstanding events and discoveries. They represent experiences which on balance have been enjoyable, rewarding, and steps toward realization.

But not all experiences are enjoyable. To partially balance the record, I include here accounts of the most miserable experiences I have had.

The following is a report of an experience with TMA-6.[1] It is my only experience with the substance; I have not been eager to try it again.

> I take 40 m.g. in a group of nine people. Dosages range from 35 m.g. to 50 m.g. As the experience grows in intensity, I feel a strong negative component developing. Several attempts of using techniques to get free of the discomfort are unsuccessful. Others are having a very enjoyable time. Two members report that it is just like MDMA.
>
> I attempt to join others in conversation. Because of my discomfort, I have a difficult time following them. In one conversation with two others, I am amazed at their sensitivity and subtlety of perception. I feel like a clod by comparison. As soon as something is mentioned that I don't grasp I blank out completely, as though all further input is hopeless until I go back and clarify what I missed. I have a difficult time expressing myself. Nothing I can say seems worthwhile. I see the great value in understanding other people's perceptions and images. I know I must try. The others are considerate and patient in helping me communicate.
>
> Despite the excited conversations that everyone else is having, which would usually draw me like a magnet, I have a powerful need to go inside. I spend time alone releasing to the experience. Although I do not break through to relief, I drain off sufficient discomfort to occasionally join the conversation. But the discomfort continues to grow.
>
> We sit down to an elaborate, beautifully prepared dinner. But my discomfort reaches such intensity I cannot sit at the table. I feel like screaming with madness. I go lie down. A female member of the group comes and puts my head in her lap. She is very comforting and I feel her deep love. She talks to me about things which start to engage my mental faculties. When she mentions that others are watching to see how I solve this problem, I realize that at least I can be better company for the others. I rejoin them, and begin to enjoy the experience.
>
> The others leave; Jean and I are spending the night with the hostess and host. I am wobbly and it is hard to keep my attention focused, but I manage to help clean up the kitchen.
>
> It feels good to get in bed, but the chemical is still driving hard. I become aware of my sexual inadequacies and selfishness. I toss and turn all night without sleeping.
>
> At seven a.m. the next morning I am somewhat rested despite no sleep. I begin to focus attention on the experience. I flow love, which leads to an enormous breakthrough. I find myself in a stout, hemispherical shell, curled up in the solid part, thoroughly walled off but absolute master within the shell. I am calling all the shots, making all of the decisions; I am in complete control. Moving out of the half-shell means becoming vulnerable, which I refuse to do. This results in my inability to hear others and share their perceptions and

their lives. I keep relationships shallow and pull away into my shell rather than become involved. I like to be to myself.

This is a great revelation; I had never seen it before. This event dissolves away my tension and I move into a state of great clarity. For the next two hours I lie and review many aspects of my life with much understanding. I see my difficulty with my son and how to improve our relationship. I gain insight into my business operation. My anger with some of the personnel and what I perceive as misdeeds are largely a projection of my unhappiness with myself. As I clear up the things that were bothering me, a gastric disturbance that has bothered me all night disappears.

The rest of the day following the experience I felt completely normal with no affect. There was not the usual post-experience elation. Instead I was very matter-of-fact, very detached. I functioned effectively as required in the moment.

The previous day I had been quite disturbed by not being able to discover what was wrong with me. The resolution occurring the morning following the experience brought much peace. I wondered if it were necessary to go through all of that anguish to find resolutions, and whether part of the discomfort might have been the result of this particular drug. But as time passed and I got further away from the experience, I remembered only the good parts and how good I felt afterwards. I am extremely grateful for this breakthrough, but am content to put this particular substance behind me.

*BOD*. This is my first trial with a new substance, BOD.[2] I take 20 m.g.; hardier souls take 25 m.g. As it gathers momentum a deep, underlying discomfort develops. While some of the positive aspects develop, like visual enhancement and appreciation of the beauty of nature, the discomfort has grown so that the beauty is marred. I am not entirely crippled; I can enjoy some things, but my attention span is very short and I cannot follow anything requiring comprehension. I have some queasiness that fades in and out over a three hour period. Listening to others becomes more and more difficult.

I lie in the sun and attempt to find the source of my discomfort, without success. The most likely source is my zeal in helping others – I am aware of their difficulties, and seem to gather them all up within myself. Then I am unable to discharge them. Nothing I have previously learned to free myself from discomfort seems to work; I have very little volition, and finally simply succumb to the experience.

After several hours, the discomfort finally drains off and I begin to enjoy the experience. Beauty returns; I feel the warmth of the group and a strong sense of Presence. Though not elated, I have a strong, powerful sense of goodness, inner strength, and solidarity.

This experience produced a powerful aftermath. Some deep inner barriers were dissolved. Although languid for a couple of days, I broke free and alertness, energy and strength became pronounced.

I functioned with ease and clarity during visits with friends and family. The ten hour drive home had all the dimensions of a true psychedelic experience, with the advantage of occurring spontaneously without effort.

Although the above experience included a great deal of discomfort, the outcome was superb. So I was anxious to try it again. Also, I was curious what effect the group made, and elected to do the next experiment in our home. I also wondered if a lighter dose would ease the discomfort. Jean did not plan to participate, but simply stand by. As luck would have it, a dear friend needed a ride to the hospital in Bishop. Jean volunteered and I was left alone.

I take 15 m.g. of BOD. It intensifies considerably in two hours. So does the feeling of squeamishness; it helps to sit outdoors in the sun.

Over the next two hours I do a great deal of searching within with the help of a mirror. The internal discomfort is present but not disturbing. I accept it, confident I will work through it. I see clearly my method of functioning is to choose a goal and plod toward it with such determination that I shut everything else out, particularly Jean.

I lie down and am gripped by fear. I realize I have not consulted my deeper self and find this prospect frightening. I open up listening to music, Stravinsky's Petrushka. As I develop the capacity to listen I am struck by the beauty, depth, variety, and creativity of the music. It is superbly engaging and beyond words to describe. Taking previous advice, I change my fear to wonder and take off on exhilarating, exciting journeys. I ask what I am afraid of; the answer is love. I find that consciously directing love requires exertion; I feel too tired to do it. I force myself, and energy begins to flow. I am hit with an enormous impact: *love is never tiring!!*

I discover my enormous need to be right, and how I love to win. This is the source of my addiction to football: I love to choose a team and exult when they win. And suffer miserably when they lose. But the bottom line is not accepting who I am.

My withdrawals fill me with energy. I am extremely intoxicated, but still manage to function. I feed our dog Spatzy, mind the stereo. When I'm up I am jittery, restless, need to pace. I go back to music. I realize I have to turn on love, keep creating it. When I stop, the uncomfortable feeling develops inside.

I flow love to other people. This is an inaccurate concept; it assumes something is wrong with other people. The world and people are already perfect. Some just don't know it. I can help the most by seeing them as they truly are.

I remember a friend telling me that when he takes LSD, the first thing he does is heal himself. Another friend said you must first love yourself. Taking their advice, as discomforts develop in my body, I flow love into them until the discomfort disappears. This is marvelous, marvelous. At one point I feel born again. But this time I am extremely grateful, glad to be alive.

I practice the meditation of watching the breath. This also is an exquisite experience. I very much feel God's presence and the wonder of the breath and being alive. Breathing connects me to eternity.

But what happens when the breath stops? This brings fear, but I remember you can learn nothing except with trust and love. I flow love and reach a state of utter stillness. I become so quiet that energy can flow in from the deep mind. This is healing, cleansing, euphoric. I cannot hold this very long, but I am able to repeat it several times. I fully appreciate the importance of reaching this quiet, still space.

I become aware that I have violated a compact I had made before taking birth this incarnation. This was to hold steady who I really am. Instead I am swayed all over the map by my own and other people's problems. I must recommit to holding reality steady; this is the best thing I can do.

The aftermath of this experience was even better than a recent powerful experience with 2C-B (following MDMA). This had more solidity, more strength, permits being more down to earth. Also, without anyone else present I maintained a constant inner dialogue, which led to a continual flow of ideation, much like LSD. I am most pleased, as I had previously attributed much of my feeling of well-being to strength gathered from others in the group.

There is a remarkable difference between the first and second trial of BOD. Part could well be the learning or growth that comes from the initial experience. The lower dose may be an important factor in maintaining volition and the ability to focus and direct the experience. In fact I was surprised to learn how important it was for me to make conscious decisions and exert the effort to love. This kept turning my experience around all day.

*Aleph 4.* I take 7 m.g. of Aleph-4[3] with Jean and three other companions. We go to one of our favorite hiking places on wooded, grassy slopes not far from the ocean. As the effect of the drug comes on I experience discomfort. This continues to grow for several hours. It feels like a solid, miserable weight in the center of my body. The discomfort reaches a peak of intensity that is most distressing. It is a heavy, dull ache that totally absorbs me. Fortunately, after a couple of hours the positive effects begin to develop, and I alternate between suffering and enjoyment. In time the enjoyment begins to outweigh the discomfort. By the time we return home in the late afternoon, I am substantially enjoying the experience.

This is a very long-acting substance, and I am unable to sleep the entire night. I keep releasing to the experience, and suddenly realize that I am the anti-Christ! I am doing horrible things to my family and to my friends, being totally absorbed in self-centeredness. I see how this interferes with learning and destroys intimacy. I get insight after insight about people that I know and how we relate. I get a large dose of my unwillingness to be considerate of others, be aware of their problems, or attempt to be of help.

I arise the next morning extremely tired. It is Father's Day and we have a date in Santa Cruz with my son and his family. I would love to stay in bed, but I know I must master my feelings and prepare for the day. The house is a mess from entertaining our guests. I clean up with great pain, forcing myself to make one move at a time. I move like a zombie, slowly and deliberately. It feels as though all previous habits have been washed away, and I have to weigh and decide each act. The amount of work seems hopeless to accomplish, but I know I must do each step, regardless of the cost. Making a deep decision to perform each act overrides the pain. Once in the car things ease up, and the day progressively gets better.

The next day at work I experience considerable undefined anxiety. At lunch I eat pizza and minestrone, which dissipates the anxiety. I understand why people each starchy foods to relieve their inner discomfort.

I felt the effects of this experience for many days. It made an enormous impact on me; it was a striking blow to my self-centeredness and self-preoccupation. A subsequent experience with a larger group repeated and intensified the discomfort without the beneficial learning, so I lost interest in this particular compound.

. . . . . . .

All of the above experiences were very valuable, and great learning experiences. But is it necessary to be so uncomfortable?

The causes of uncomfortable experiences are hotly debated. There are persons who claim that some of the new substances are toxic. Others state that we all have different body chemistries and some drugs do not sit as well with us as others; different people can react differently to a particular drug. Or we may encounter deeply buried, painful material.

I have never ingested ibogaine, but I have interviewed several who have. They hold ibogaine in high regard as a powerful agent of learning and change.

After my experiences with BOD, I am tempted to conclude that a powerful agent for change is the uncomfortable feelings that may occur. One is so miserable that you can't help wondering, what is wrong with me? And you are willing to look for any solution. This includes a thorough review of anything you might be doing wrong in your life, and an exhaustive search for anything that might ease the discomfort.

I confess to a powerful disposition to make all experiences meaningful. The fact that they are unpleasant does not necessarily mean that they are not valuable. In fact, the discomfort most generally arises from the resistance to experiencing painful material. So if such material is successfully encountered and resolved, there is a great gain in psychic freedom and well-being.

It is an important part of Tibetan Buddhist practice to use adversity as a means to the path of enlightenment. Alan Wallace, in his book *A Passage From Solitude*, presents Seven Point Mind Training as he has translated it from ancient Tibetan texts and received from oral transmissions. He states that the third point is perhaps the best-known aspect of this training, and is entitled Using Unfavorable Circumstances As Aids to Awakening.[4]

I am grateful for the inner searching I have done, and the growth and development that resulted. And if it took considerable discomfort to propel me into the need to search, so be it. The results are salutary.

But having once covered that ground, and learning what was offered, I see no need to go that route again. I have learned that the appropriate use of love is the most effective learning aid. I believe this tool can be used with more benign substances.

Of course pleasant substances do not guarantee pleasant experiences, as who knows what may be lurking in the unconscious, or what the Supreme Teacher has in store for us to learn? But I don't need to load the dice against me, and shall probably not try BOD again, even though it worked well for others. Fortunately there are a lot of new, exciting substances to investigate further.

### Chapter 7 Notes


1. Shulgin, A. T. & Shulgin, A. *PIHKAL, A Chemical Love Story.* Berkeley, California: Transform Press, 1991, pp. 876-9.
2. Ibid., pp. 492-6.
3. Ibid., pp. 468-9.
4. Wallace, Alan B. *A Passage from Solitude.* Ithaca, N.Y.: Snow Lion Publications, 1992, pp. 61-72

# Chapter 8
# Low Doses

There are a number of experienced experts in the field of psychedelics who recommend not fooling around with low doses. Andrew Weil, in his chapter in Lester Grinspoon's and James Bakalar's book *Psychedelic Reflections*,[1] states:

> Half doses of psychedelics seldom work. They are more likely to produce restlessness and dysphoria than the reactions we seek. Several times I have been in small groups where one member only wanted to take a half dose. That desire expresses a reluctance to make the necessary commitment to the group, to the day, to the experience. My advice in that circumstance is take the drug or not, rather than go it halfway.

Terence McKenna, renowned expert on psychoactive plant materials, also offers similar advice. If you want the real experience, you have to be sure to take enough. Otherwise you may slither around in the nether regions.

I know others who share the same view. Their idea is to blast themselves into transcendental levels by taking a goodly amount of a powerful sacrament. I notice, however, when the experiences are over, that this world is often an uncomfortable place for them. The paradise they experience under the glory of the high doses is in sharp contrast to what appears to be the hum-drum, dreary, everyday world.

I have never been able to validate personally this information on high doses. For many years the onset of my psychedelic experience has been quite uncomfortable. Very often, increasing the dose level simply increased the agony and the length of time I would struggle until I broke through into a remarkable space.

So my experience has been different. I suspect that those who like me have poor self-images, are carrying heavy loads of anger or bitterness, or do not sufficiently trust life may have a more difficult time breaking through into those wonderful transcendental levels. However it may be, I think it worthwhile to examine the other side of the coin and look at possible advantages of taking smaller amounts.

Some of the best information that I have accumulated regarding the efficacy of low doses comes from a couple who are both very competent psychologists. On one occasion when they visited us, I was surprised at the very small amount of substance they ingested. Despite this small amount, they both had wonderful experiences.

In discussing the topic, they say that the reason most people don't wish to take low doses is that they don't care for the uncomfortable feelings which ensue. These feelings are, however, extremely important. They are precisely those feelings that are interfering with our life, and need to be resolved. Therefore it is worthwhile to experience them, confront them, and resolve them.

This sounded like excellent advice to me. So I followed their instructions, and for several journeys I used smaller amounts. I found what they said to be quite true. The feelings were uncomfortable, but I soon realized that they are my feelings, they are an important part of me, and it was important for me to be at home with them. In fact, it seemed clear that these feelings are the source of my discomfort in journeys and in day-to-day life.

I willingly confronted them and stayed with them, giving them my full attention until they resolved themselves. This process usually started with me recognizing that I was uncomfortable. Most of the time it was a vague, sluggish feeling that I did not specifically recognize. As I held my attention steadily on it, it would become more clear. Often I would begin to understand what my true feeling was, what were my true desires, or what I was doing wrong with my life or relationships. With recognition, my feelings would begin to release and simply float away. I found that as I worked through them and released them, my feeling of well-being began to rise, as did my energy level. As I continued to work on these feelings, I found myself getting into the same valuable spaces that I cherished with the larger doses.

In the end, I concluded with experiences just as profound with the lower doses as I did with larger amounts. But there was a very significant gain: I had resolved a lot of interior debris, so that I felt much more at peace with myself, and the after-effects of the experience stayed with me in a rewarding way for a much longer period of time. Also, since I had learned to deal with my feelings, I became much more adept at handling them as they came up in daily situations.

Here are some excerpts from a couple of experiences to illustrate how this has worked for me. Both experiences are with 2C-T-7,[2] for which I consider 20 m.g. to be a full dose:

> Jean takes 15 m.g., I take 12 m.g. of 2C-T-7. I am following the suggestion that it may be more effective to take lighter amounts and work through what I encounter on that level.
>
> The intensity is growing at 1-1/2 hours, and I develop some unpleasant feelings. I'm not concerned; I'll take what I get and see what I can learn.
>
> Going into meditation is very pleasant; the discomfort clears up. I enjoy sitting quietly and holding my mind still. However, as soon as I stop concentrating the discomfort returns. I'm not able to pinpoint the source. If I focus on appreciation or love everything turns bright and beautiful. But I prefer to hold still and see if things won't turn out good on their own. I want to feel there is a beneficent Source underlying everything, without me having to do anything about it. I have intimations of this, but I can't get clearly into it.
>
> I think about loving myself, and look into a mirror. I have a very amusing experience with a surge of good feelings as I see how much I love myself in a completely self-centered sense. I feel this guy I am looking at is hot shit. Part of me feels wiser, smarter than anybody(!!). It feels very good, because I have never before allowed myself to see my inner inflation.
>
> Meditating, I encounter lots of stress resulting from my always setting up goals and objectives and putting a lot of investment into accomplishing them. It feels wonderful to let all my investments go and simply relax.
>
> Despite occasionally rising into beautiful experiences and good feelings, I always fall back into a gnawing, deep discomfort. I lie down and relax completely; this releases the discomfort. I realize that I am a failure. I look at this in all its aspects. I feel how powerful is my drive to win. Now it is a great re-

lief to be willing to fail in whatever I attempt. Also, it feels great to indulge in my feelings, free of scruples. I have always controlled my feelings through rational decisions, and now I enjoy indulging them completely, despite inappropriate consequences. I discharge a lot of the discomfort.

I want to be in God's presence. Again I look to see if I can feel this Presence without me conjuring up anything. I want to feel God's love for me as I am. Immediately the question arises in my mind whether I accept others the way that they are. I see that I care for people based largely on what they accomplish. I spend some time feeling what it's like to care for others only for their essence. I think of several persons I know for whom this is difficult, but it is rewarding to work on it.

After a goodly amount of inner work, it is a welcome change to sit on the deck and drink in the surrounding landscape. Release of repressed feelings cleared my mind and raised my energy level, permitting a marvelous contemplative state. I spend a lot of time looking at my relationship with Jean. I see that when I doubt if she is an appropriate partner, I am making her less. As I drop the judgment, I can feel the expansion of her being. When I turn my attention to her well-being, it raises my own level of enjoyment.

While my feeling tone has improved during the day, I can't completely get away from an inner discomfort. I decide to abandon my previous position of just experiencing what's there, and go into an active procedure. I do the loving-kindness meditation, drawing love in from the cosmos on the in-breath, and radiating it out to all around me on the out-breath. This raises the level of joy, despite producing a little tension in my body. As I keep this up, my energy level goes up considerably, along with my feeling of being "on top". I feel some inner hurts, and it is a marvelous release to draw love into them and heal them. I am healing myself, which seems to be the most important thing anyone can do. After thirty to forty minutes of this, everything around me is lit up with energy and love. I am in a whole new state, enormously enjoying the surrounding beauty and wonder. This marvelous feeling stays with me the rest of the day.

Here is another experience on 15 m.g. of 2C-T-7:

I am aware of being very forward with Debra, a double widow I met at a family picnic at the ocean. I realized I talked too much beyond her frame of reference; I must be much more aware of where people are. Also, I had a hard time withholding judgment as I became aware of her nasty side. I am very troubled about how to deal with this. The only answer is love, despite how hard it is.

Jean wants to hear the Moody Blues. I find it obnoxious. Then I thought, if I cared for her, I should be able to share her enjoyment. I discover this to be true.

I went through many realizations about love. With true love, you don't mind the pain; it's worth it. For real love, anything is worth it. This is a profound realization. I am able to get deeply into the dynamic of love; this is most gratifying.

I lie on the couch and continue the inward journey, which feels very good. It is clear that the whole point is to be with the inner teacher. I come closer and closer to being able to experience the true essence of another person, which seems to me to be the best resolution of judgments.

I find myself as a baby in my mother's arms, in bed. I experience a wonderful feeling of peace. I see that much of my life, including a lot of my snuggling time with Jean, is an effort to get back to this feeling of peace where I feel completely cared for and don't have to do anything. I can see why she resents it. I decide it's time to grow up and take responsibility for myself, so I get up.

I feel very alert, energized, thoroughly intoxicated, but in excellent command of my body. I can't see any detrimental effect from having had a little breakfast (we usually fast on experience days so as not to dilute the chemical), and my innards are more comfortable. The latter part of the afternoon is the best part of the experience. I am learning how to be with my Teacher, discovering a variety of noteworthy things. I see that this is a most valuable state for everyone to arrive at, and I shouldn't spoil their initiation into it by saying anything about it. It is between each individual and God, and everything is there for the person who wants it. I am more convinced than ever that my interest in saving the world is an escape from my own personal growth. It is most important to develop oneself and one's family and home.

At one point, wondering how to turn anger into love, I see that they are opposites and inexorably linked. If I can intensify anger, I can also intensify love. By becoming aware of the depth of my anger, the whole sky turns into the brilliant light of love. Incredible.

The universe is there to carry out whatever I wish to do with love. Lapsing into intellectualization cuts off the experience. It requires being totally present, holding the mind still and steady and free of conceptualizing. Then reality reveals itself. I have a remarkable time seeing how much reality I can allow to manifest. The intensity of love, beauty, and meaning continues to grow with attention and gratitude.

I find I still have areas to resolve with Jean, but I'm learning more about how to do this all the time. It's a fascinating process, and I am eagerly pursuing it day by day.

An experience with Jean and me and another couple is an excellent illustration of the use of small doses. Here are some highlights from the experience we shared together:

We took what would ordinarily be one full dose for a single person of this particular substance, and divided it four ways. Much to our amazement, it turned out to be a full-blown experience for all of us! We were all elated with the experience, and enjoyed much beauty, euphoria, and binding love among the group of us. We particularly appreciated the splendor of our surroundings. We agreed that it was one of our best experiences in recent times.

At one point in the experience, I suggested that we all be still together, and gave a short guided meditation to induce the stillness. The instructions were very similar to that for watching the breath as in Vipassana meditation, with the added comment of being aware of why we were doing this, to invite the Presence. Our patient willingness to continue the process is a demonstration of our desire, a desire that if sufficiently expressed would undoubtedly be answered.

Everyone reported afterwards that this practice opened up a rewarding level of encounter. One said that it set the tone for the day, giving the appropriate direction to the experience. Everyone present was highly motivated to have as profound an experience of the Divine as possible, and found the stillness an effective entry into contact with the Numinous.

In mid-afternoon I was feeling some heaviness. I debated whether I should supplement, but I chose not to. When the others decided to go for a walk, I opted to stretch out in a lounge chair on the deck. I went into meditation, and found that as I did so the heaviness began to clear up. I continued this process and found myself moving into a deeper experience of God's Presence. The joy of His love and the wonder of being the instrument for His love welled up in me. Once I began to move into this space, I was content to sit there by the hour and simply enjoy the wonder, the joy, the beauty, and the marvelous grace that was coming to me.

One member of the group moved into realms of such beauty it was impossible for her to behold. I don't believe she had previously experienced such profound levels of love and beauty.

But then the experience became almost too much. She found it better to walk around, observing the wonder of the late afternoon sunset. This contact with her surroundings maintained stability. She found that the experience came in waves, and at the peak of the waves she would feel marvelous ecstasy and enjoyment. However the next wave would bring anxiety and she would have to work through that again.

While this was going on, I lay on a mattress on the side of the house facing the mountains. I closed my eyes, and although I was feeling good, I felt tired. I allowed myself to sink into the tiredness, and told myself I was willing to die. Simply letting go completely, relaxing completely, was a most enjoyable experience. After a while I felt myself in the womb with the most satisfying feeling of not having to do anything. I felt like everything was being taken care of, and I had no responsibilities whatever. This was a very blissful feeling, and I enjoyed it enormously. For quite a long time I felt like Penfield's mouse[3] that held its foot on the pedal which stimulated the pleasure center in its brain. I could have gone on for hours and hours.

That evening food was a treat. We thoroughly enjoyed each other's company. A great bonding had grown among us, and although we had always been good friends, this was carried forward into a new dimension of realization. So this experience with an almost insignificant amount of substance turned out to be one of the very best!

I was very glad that I hadn't taken the supplement, because it felt very good to reach the same space under my own power. As I described it to the others, it seems necessary to develop a God muscle. If we simply allow ourselves to get into these spaces by taking more substance, then we are not developing what it takes within ourselves to accomplish this on our own. I was very grateful for doing it this way, and felt much stronger inside.

Today, four days after this low dose experience, I climbed to a very high place on a very steep mountain and was in remarkably good physical condition. I never had to gulp for air or be out of breath or be tired as I was only the week before. I am at the peak of my physical condition, and I am enjoying this climb more than any I can remember in many, many years. This certainly is the way to live!!

I do not mean to imply by the above discussion that low doses are necessarily superior to high doses. They each have their place. In fact, I have often found that supplementing with additional chemical in the middle of an experience has been very salutary, freeing up uncomfortable stuck areas and allowing me to penetrate more deeply into other levels of awareness.

And sometimes not. Sometimes the additional amount has simply increased agitation and tension. As described in several reports in this writing, I often found it more rewarding to stick with a smaller amount and confront and resolve the feelings involved. This led to a freeing up and a breakthrough to another level. The push of a higher dose can override one's ability to stay focused on the feelings until they are resolved.

Many prefer the higher dose levels in order to reach transcendental levels of awareness. There is absolutely no question that attaining such states is one of the most prized achievements of humankind. It has no equal, and is often a life-changing experience. One accomplished spiritual leader once said to me, "Millions would give most anything they have just to know that such experiences are possible. Thousands of others would gladly die to have such an experience". To reach such a level of awareness must certainly be the first order of business for any individual seeking spiritual fulfillment.

But achieving such levels does not guarantee resolving life's problems or maintaining high states of realization. I suspect that lower doses are avoided because of the uncomfortable feelings. I offer here evidence that dealing with such feelings can be very productive in improving one's life situation, and is a course worth considering.

For well-balanced development, both high and low doses have their appropriate application. Sherry Anderson and Patricia Hopkin, in their well-researched and beautifully written book *The Feminine Face of God*, cover the issue of balanced development this way: "We believe that there are two aspects of being in the sacred garden. One part comes through receptivity through grace ... We can prepare for this, but how and when it happens is not within our control."

"The other part requires choice, an act of conscious intention to embody the sacred in our everyday life. This means that we bring our spiritual insights into every aspect of our lives – when we chop carrots for dinner, drive on the freeway, confer with our colleagues, and play with our children."

"Choice lies at the heart of the matter, because even if you have not had a direct experience of the divine, once you make a conscious choice to act on what you *do* know, the process of spiritual maturing begins."[4]

They amplify this statement with a relevant note: "It seems important to add that someone who can access refined states of consciousness is not necessarily spiritually mature ... the capacity for mystical states of consciousness is not always an indication of spiritual maturity. Spiritual maturity as we define it is the choice to live out of that consciousness in our ordinary moments."[5]

An excellent last word on the choice of dose level comes from a statement by a very good and quite knowledgeable friend: "The issue is not whether to take a high dose or a low dose, but to take a *useful* dose".

### Chapter 8 Notes

1. Lester Grinspoon and James B. Bakalar, editors. *Psychedelic Reflections*. New York: Human Sciences Press, Inc., 1983, p. 123.
2. Shulgin, A. T. & Shulgin, A. *PIHKAL, A Chemical Love Story*. Berkeley, California: Transform Press, 1991, pp. 567-71.

3. Dr. Wilder Penfield at the Montreal Neurological Institute is well known for his work of mapping the brain by electrical prospecting. By implanting electrodes in the brains of mice, he discovered a "pleasure point". Mice preferred to stimulate this pleasure point by stepping on a foot pedal rather than eat or engage in sex.
4. Sherry Ruth Anderson and Patricia Hopkins. *The Feminine Face of God.* New York: Bantam Books, 1991, p. 102.
5. Ibid. p. 232.

# Chapter 9
# Family

One of the great joys that Jean and I have experienced is sharing MDMA with our family. We found special pleasure in drawing closer in love and understanding to our relatives. First we introduced our daughter Dede (Jean's daughter, whom I adopted after we married), and then other family members. Several proved to be gifted travelers. Details of some of our experiences together follow:

*Dede.* I first met Dede when she was ten years old. I was accompanying some friends to visit Dede's mother for the first time. Dede met us on the outside steps in the court of their apartment house. Slim, extremely cute and personable, I hoped she looked a lot like her mother.

After Jean and I were married, Dede and I had our problems. Jean had previously focused her entire attention on Dede, and provided her with everything within reason. Dede very much resented my intrusion into this very nice setup, which diverted Jean's attention to me. For several years we had an armed truce. Each morning I would come down the hall, and Dede would step out of her room with a sullen look on her face. I greeted her as cheerily as I could, but most of the time got a barely audible response.

One of the greatest moments of my life was several years later, when Dede was moving to her own apartment and Jean and I were preparing to move to the high desert. I was in her room with her, a flamboyantly decorated room alive with color and new age posters. This was her private space where she was free to express herself in any way she wished. Many of her secret longings, as well as her artistic talent, were splashed on the walls.

We were discussing our impending separation. Dede said to me, "Dad, I want you to know that all these last few years when you've been telling me things, I pretended not to listen. But I heard every word and I knew you were right, and they have helped me a lot."

I was quite shaken by this announcement, and overcome with tears. I have a hard time not crying as I write this.

Jean and I shared MDMA with Dede the day after her 19th birthday.

> As soon as the experience develops to full intensity, Dede becomes aware of the way she is treating her body. She finds that she is drinking too much alcohol and not getting enough sleep. This is impressed upon her time and again.
>
> We have excellent communication among the three of us, with the marvelous freedom from defensiveness so characteristic of this substance. We end the day with excellent bonding.

Her second trial was a year later, in the company of other close relatives. We are in a condominium overlooking the ocean at San Clemente.

Dede has been suffering for some time from stomach problems, which her doctor has diagnosed as spastic colon. She is under a lot of tension from a number of changes taking place in her life. Her boyfriend is moving to San Diego to go to school, and she will soon be leaving her apartment for a new one.

In thirty-five minutes we are all well into the experience and enjoying it immensely. The ocean is a wonderful stabilizer and source of inspiration. Everyone's voice, face, skin soften. All of Dede's stomach pains disappear. She feels free of pain and tension for the first time in months. She watches the breakers, seeing them as long smiles, and the ocean saying, "Come play with me!" She writes some poetry. We are all having an outstanding time.

After the supplement, Dede says that she has never felt better in her whole life. She is very grateful for the experience. One person suggests looking down on our bodies, and if we notice any tension or pain, heal it. It works!

I find the ocean and heavy surf a great stimulus to exalted thoughts – the timelessness, feeling of eternity, the marvelous state of the world, the hope for mankind, the wonder of these materials and those that make them possible. There is a superb feeling of centeredness.

It is an enormous grace to have our family drawn close together in such a satisfying, euphoric experience. It turned out to be Dede's last experience for several years. She found that leaving us after being so closely bonded was quite painful, and didn't care to go through the distress of separation again.

*Manuel and Selma.* One couple in our family is especially interesting. My relative Manuel is an extremely open, good-natured, life-affirming person. Over the years he has followed my work with great interest, and had several very rewarding LSD experiences with Al Hubbard.

Selma is German-born, and moved to the United States after marrying an American officer, whom she later divorced. She is very attractive, very bright and sensitive, and fun-loving. She and Manuel have an ideal marriage, in that they are very much in love and thoroughly support each other. Selma has at times a sharp manner of expressing herself, which has been a bit difficult for some of the rest of us to accommodate. However, we have all grown by accepting her and by developing the inner strength to not let her criticisms, real or inferred, bother us.

Selma is quite a perfectionist. She is also very accomplished, so that whatever she tries turns out well. She was an excellent artist, and made a living by making rapid, cute, inexpensive paintings. She gave this up when she married Manuel. She is a gourmet cook, and her home is outstandingly decorated. She and Manuel travel a great deal, and they have filled their home with beautiful art objects. Unfortunately Selma puts herself under a great deal of tension, so that she has suffered from chronic pains in the abdomen for many years.

Eight years before the arrival of MDMA in our life, we thought an experience with LSD might relieve her stomach pains. Unfortunately, we did not handle the experience well. We drove to Death Valley, which in those days was a favorite way to savor the sacraments. We learned much later that many people do not relish being cooped up in a car for hours under these circumstances. Also, there were several people in our party, so that Selma felt under pressure to perform. We did not pick up her discomfort, so did not give her adequate attention. Selma found her pain heightened, not only during the experience but for several weeks afterward as well. Her lack of further interest was quite understandable.

So we were rather surprised when ten years later Selma became interested in our descriptions of MDMA, and wished to participate.

Our first journey with Manuel and Selma was at Christmas at our home in the high desert. A younger couple to whom we are related also joined us.

> Selma has a rather difficult entry, feeling a lot of resistance, inability to concentrate and slight nausea. She feels somewhat better as the experience develops. She is a good sport and takes the supplement despite her discomfort. We all move into a warm, close space and feel more and more alive. Except for Selma, we are enjoying the experience enormously and are very grateful to be together. Selma's state improves, which deepens the sharing and the bonding. The next day she has opened up a lot, and tells us a great deal about the hardships of her life in Germany during World War II. It was always a scramble to get food, and the Russian soldiers were aggressive, primitive peasants. She was in some very difficult situations with them when they took over Berlin, and she survived by her guts and her wits.

It was over a year before this same group came together for a second trial. It was heartening that it came at Selma's request, despite the fact that she had previously experienced a lot of resistance which manifested as dizziness, feelings of faintness, and unpleasantness.

What was fascinating to me was that none of these previous symptoms showed up in Selma's second experience. Despite it being a year later, she took off from where she had left off previously, and moved into a very enjoyable and fruitful experience. This dynamic has shown up a number of times in subsequent experiences with people. More than with any other substance I have observed, it seems as though they start from where they left off before. The amount of elapsed time between experiences does not seem to be a major factor. This is a characteristic that very much warrants specific investigation. The report of our second experience follows:

> This turned out to be a most rewarding day for all of us. We were able to perceive the best qualities in each other, and as we verbalized our views, our self-esteem, acceptance, and level of love and bonding rose to enormous proportions. We were able to turn our attention to very specific family problems which under ordinary circumstances would be very difficult to discuss. But here, engrossed in love and with no trace of defensiveness, we could share our perceptions freely, insightfully, and without rancor, leading to much heightened understanding and closeness. But best of all, the inner good feelings kept growing and growing, until we were filled with enormous gratitude to be with each other and feel the love that we all shared. What a magnificent contribution to our family!

*Judith.* One of the most remarkable people in my life is my beloved aunt Judith. From when my brother and I were small kids, we loved to bask in her radiance. She is a very bright, delightfully outgoing person, with sharp, penetrating perception. She sees with crystal clarity what is right and what is wrong, and has very little tolerance for those who sluff off. And she is an outstandingly giving person. At the slightest hint that someone she knows may be suffering from some discomfort, she is immediately there with hot chicken soup, blintzes, or a batch of cookies. Being an outstanding cook, any goodies she shows up with are always welcome.

When my mother died in 1956, Judith and her husband, Nathan, moved to Roswell, New Mexico, to live with my Dad. A few years later Nathan died of Parkinson's disease, his last years made much more pleasant by Judith's scrupulous care. She made an agreement to stay with my father and look after him until he passed away.

Any person would be extremely lucky to have Judith look after them. She is thoughtful, compassionate, understanding, and absolutely tireless and unselfish in ministering to the needs of others. My Dad certainly had it good. He had excellent meals just as he liked them, warm companionship, and could bask in Judith's delightful presence.

It wasn't always easy. Dad was demanding and unappreciative, like a lot of us, and could be quite cruel in his negligence of Judith and her needs. And as for we brothers! We were delighted that someone so capable was taking care of Dad, so that it didn't disrupt our busy lives. This went over with Judith like a lead balloon!

But she didn't suffer in silence. She spoke her mind to us time and again, and we began to wake up and lift some of the burden of looking after Dad's welfare. But it was not enough and too late. After Dad died, it took a while for Judith to overcome the bitterness. But she is a very forgiving person, so that in time she dropped her resentments and we could all be friends.

While Judith was looking after Dad, I kept them abreast of my work in psychedelic research. Judith had her hands full, and paid little attention. After Dad's death, she moved to Tucson to be near her two sons and their families, and to do what she could for their welfare. She always had had a great deal of respect for me, so now she became much more interested in my work. After a few years she felt that she had done all that she could to help her family, and was satisfied with their well-being and self-sufficiency. So she could take the chance of having her mind altered, even if it was irreversible.

She had heard quite a bit about MDMA, and this seemed the ideal substance to introduce her to this new world. After Dad died she had become quite close to Manuel and Selma and to us. We agreed to share a journey together. So this is how a 79 year old woman undertook her first experience with MDMA.

It was a beautiful setting, in a smartly appointed home. We and our hosts, Manuel and Selma, were already very close from sharing our love with each other.

> We all take 120 m.g. of MDMA. It comes on delightfully gentle and euphoric. We are all in a most enjoyable space, thoroughly appreciating each other. As it reaches full intensity, it opens a floodgate of communication for Judith. Living alone, and not having intimate friends in Tucson, and not being too well understood by her family, she had withheld an enormous amount of thoughts and feelings. Now it all comes gushing out.
>
> She is so intoxicated she slightly slurs her speech, but continues almost nonstop. As I observe her, she is like a powerful, bright, radiant light. There is a marvelous, luminous quality to her being; it is a joy to be in her presence. Her mind is sharp and clear; she allows absolutely no wishy-washiness to obscure her vision, no matter what the cost to herself.

She has been very hurt by the misunderstandings that have developed within her family in Tucson. Judith observes everything in an extremely clear light, and immediately expresses what she observes. She does not see that for people without this clarity of vision, her remarks can be very scathing. She recounts at great length the faults with various individuals and their unthinking, often unintelligent actions. And how much she has been hurt by their reactions, which have included disbelief, opposition, rejection. Having a very strong disposition herself, she doesn't understand how much people are hurt when their delicate egos are threatened, and how powerful are their defenses.

It is a great relief to Judith to be carefully listened to, and she unburdens a great deal of her resentments. Then through our general discussion, she begins to appreciate that others may have a different viewpoint, to which they are entitled. And she begins to see that real love and concern requires honoring others, and being careful not to confront them with information they are not really seeking. Fortunately our own group, with our deep love for Judith, is a marvelous example of how caring people communicate. She is a very sensitive person, and deeply feels the love from us all. As we talk and explore different aspects of relationships, and as the experience develops, we continue to draw closer and closer. It reaches the point where she experiences love far greater than at any time previously.

Judith is an extremely honest person. More than anyone I have seen, she was determined to take the lessons she had learned and apply them directly in her life. She lost no time in talking to her sons, her daughters-in-law, and her grandchildren. There was still a lot to work out for real understanding, and of course it is difficult with a one-sided approach. But her understanding of the dynamics between her and her family grew rapidly, as well as her self-confidence and contentment with herself. She felt her MDMA experience was an enormous grace, and completely changed her life. No one I have known has worked with more determination to bring her life into accord with the teachings of her experience.

Judith has had MDMA two additional times. Each time she has honestly examined her situation and has seen more clearly. She has come to realize that some situations cannot be resolved, and not everyone wishes to take her advice. She has learned to offer it when it is wanted. But she has come to peace with her own situation, and no longer allows others to dictate her well-being. Everyone in our family who knows of her experiences greatly admires her courage and her honesty, and her desire to be the best possible person that she can be. And every one of us consider it a great honor when we can spend time with her.

. . . . . . .

Repeated experiences with family members continued to heighten our bonding and the joy of being with each other. This has brought us full appreciation for what a family can mean to each other.

While this same bonding and appreciation grows from sharing with good friends, I am drawn to feel that a primitive, basic requirement is fulfilled in pulling family members together. It is as though learning to be close and acknowledging and supporting each other starts with the family. It may be my Jewish heritage and the emphasis that Jewish people put on family. And often it is hardest to develop intimacy with those to whom we are closest. What is certain is that the results of this approach are very satisfying.

# Chapter 10
# Good Friends Along the Way I

Some of the richest rewards that ensue from pursuing psychedelic exploration with close friends comes from the deep, richly satisfying relationships that develop.

Relationships deepen by way of a two-pronged dynamic. First there is the clearing of individual beings – the dissolving away of repressed material, the recognizing and dropping of outdated concepts and habits, the dropping of defenses. This opens the space among participants and allows an increasing intimacy. As the barriers dissolve, the energy radiated from each person increases. The combined linking of these radiant sources yields a strong energy field, a field of bonding love that supports and strengthens each one in the group.

The other prong consists in exploring new areas of consciousness, which brings into the group a wealth of new information. Each of course apprehends this in his/her own, unique way. The sharing and discussion of such discoveries leads to greater clarification and understanding in each member of the group. The issues go all the way from personal dynamics to the nature of God and how one achieves and maintains transcendence.

This chapter and the following one are devoted to material gathered from explorations and exchanges with good friends.

## *Duncan*

One of the fascinating, significant figures in the early days of psychedelics was a psychologist in Canada. In the early 1950's, when LSD was first introduced, investigators were busily engaged in determining the nature of this substance and the results it produced. The medical establishment rapidly arrived at the conclusion that LSD produces a state which mimicked psychosis, and named it a psychotomimetic.

Fortunately there were others who because of some combination of having an appropriate world view, being completely at peace with themselves, having a lively curiosity and a willingness to relinquish preconceived ideas, were able to move into completely different areas of experience with these substances.

Duncan was one of these. Although a brilliant psychologist, he was an extremely lovable, fun-loving person. When he and Al Hubbard came together there was instant rapport. They recognized each other as scoundrels and explorers, and immediately formed a deep alliance. The following excerpts of a letter from Duncan to Al gives the flavor of their relationship:

> Hello you old goat!
>
> Whose old uncle forgets him and never, never writes him a letter? My uncle Al – that's who.

What are they doing to you these days that you neglect your fat nephew? I've been watching the incoming mail, meeting all the aircraft and reading the police news regularly in hopes that I'd catch some glimpse of a letter from you, yourself, or your name in headlines. However, despite my vigilance there hasn't been the slightest indication that you are still alive. If I didn't know that it would take a battalion of enraged grizzly bears to do you in, I'd have been so worried I wouldn't sleep by now.

There is another picture that floats through my mind however – in fact a whole series of pictures of Al basking in the sunshine of some Pacific Isle, watching ball games in Witchita, catching huge fish off Boca Grande and generally living a life of idle bliss ...

How's about a few lines of communication to let me know if we still fly the same flag – and what the latest developments have been.

All the very best of good wishes. May the sound of police whistles cease to annoy you and become music to your ears.

Love,
Dunc.

With Al's companionship, Duncan freely explored vast areas of consciousness with wise comprehension. Hubbard was fond of carrying around a little tape recorder playing back a statement that Duncan pronounced during one of his explorations. It ended with the statement: "The true meaning of life is so simple that scientists will never discover it."

I heard many stories about Duncan from Hubbard. Duncan had many gifts and talents, including the Irish ability to eloquently describe the multifarious situations he often found himself in. And his ability to creatively resolve them.

Duncan was quite enthused about the worlds that LSD opened up and the enormous potential such experiences held for the betterment of mankind. Consequently at one psychological meeting where he presented a paper, he recommended that LSD should be available in gum-ball machines in every drugstore. While current American society is shocked by such a suggestion, it must be remembered that at that time LSD was being used very successfully in several areas in Canada as a treatment for alcoholism. Saskatchewan was one of the few places in time and geography when the man on the street recognized LSD as a valuable medicine, and that its use was the most effective treatment for alcoholism then known. As alcoholism was quite a scourge in those cold, northern climates where winters left little opportunity for entertainment, cures were very much appreciated by suffering families.

I looked forward very much to meeting Duncan, and one summer afternoon in Vancouver I had the opportunity. I was visiting with Al and Rita, and was advised that Duncan would soon be arriving for a visit.

We were aware when his car entered the parking lot of the apartment house, and we opened the door of Hubbard's fourth floor apartment. We could hear Duncan tromping up the stairs. As he turned around the last landing, I got my first glimpse of him.

Duncan was a short, stocky man, with short arms. Wearing a sleeveless sportshirt appropriate for the warm, sunny day, he was flamboyantly climbing the stairs, swinging his arms in a way that revealed the engaging movement of his exposed elbows. A happy, fun-loving grin lighted up his face. Grasped in one hand was a large, green peyote button, which he stuffed into his mouth from time to time and chewed happily.

Duncan had also heard of me, and after being introduced, the first thing he did was to offer me a bite of his button. I accepted, and found much to my surprise that it didn't taste nearly as bad as I had been led to believe.

That evening we went out to dine at Hubbard's favorite place reserved for the most prominent visitors, the Vancouver Yacht Club. It was a decorous setting, and an ideal place to get acquainted while simultaneously enjoying an excellently served gourmet meal.

I was thoroughly engaged by the wonderful stories Duncan was sharing. I had had such a small amount of the peyote that I never felt it. So imagine my surprise when I looked at the lush carpet and found all the designs raised in three-D, and with glowing colors! I was delighted, as this was the first time in my life I have observed visual effects without any feeling of ingesting a drug. I felt only the well-being of superb companionship.

Duncan was telling us where he got the peyote. At that time it was possible to procure it from a source in Texas. He and his friends had chipped in and ordered a gunny-sack full. Not sure how it would be accepted by Canadian law, they elected to store it under the front porch of the home of one member of the group. Here they felt it would be safe; this person's father was the local sheriff. They never bothered to tell him about it.

Duncan played an active role in Saskatchewan as a therapist and guide in the experimental use of LSD with alcoholic subjects. Working with other hospital staff, encouraging results were achieved. Duncan wrote a most knowledgeable handbook about the informed use of LSD in a therapeutic setting. Despite it being written before 1960, it is still the most comprehensive, thorough, and knowledgeable treatment of the subject in print today, other than Stan Grof's volume *LSD Psychotherapy*.[1] The work accomplished in the last three decades by other therapists (who have had to work underground because of our repressive drug laws) confirms the accuracy of the information presented.

At one point there was a debate as to whether or not LSD is addicting. Duncan was sure that it was not, so in order to prove it, he and his supervising psychiatrist took it every day as they sat with experimental subjects. At the end of 30 days he declared that there was no change in his ordinary functioning.

However, some of the authorities at the treatment hospital declared that he was addicted because he was taking it every day. So they demanded that he and his supervisor stop taking it. They stopped, and exhibited no adverse effects. Duncan was a bit sad at being deprived of the opportunity to partake.

I had the good fortune to share a few experiences with Duncan, and found him extremely sensitive, aware, helpful, and companionable. He was one of the easiest persons to love I have ever met. I grew very fond of him. I regret the distance that separates us, and the exigencies in life that have widened the separation. I often wonder what has happened to him, and what he is doing now. I believe he retired to a home in Mexico. If he has his way, I am sure that he is sharing a peyote button or two with some new-found friend.

## *Jeffrey*

Jeffrey was a long time friend, and one of the most interesting people that I have known. He was a teacher of religion and philosophy at one of our well-known universities, and always had a deep interest in the mystical and the occult. For years he had meetings in his home, inviting outstanding personages to address or demonstrate to a group of friends who shared his interests.

Jeffrey was thrilled to learn that there were substances available which could provide entry to the states with which he was so enamored. He became one of the first volunteers, and thoroughly enjoyed his experiences.

Besides his teaching occupation, Jeffrey was also a trained architect, and had designed and built a very beautiful home. There is one additional area that I considered him a complete standout.

One of the ways that Al Hubbard had taught us to prepare people for the psychedelic experience was to give them some inhalations of Maduna's mixture of carbon dioxide and oxygen.[2] I personally had derived a great deal from this procedure. It was a marvelous abreactor, and for me always released an enormous charge of repressed anger. Despite the fact that the release was always freeing and exhilarating, I always approached the experience with a great deal of anxiety. While most people who went through our program at the Foundation derived considerable benefit, it was such a drastic and dramatic procedure that no one underwent it eagerly.

Jeffrey was quite an exception. He loved it. He would take an enormous number of breathes – up to 50, whereas most would release their inhibitions with 15 to 20. But his experiences were always exalted. He would have intense and varied imagery, often of outstanding architectural forms. He always returned to normal consciousness with a bit of sadness at leaving such a wonderful world, yet very grateful for the opportunity to spend some time there.

As we got busy with our work at the Foundation, I lost track of Jeffrey. He developed some heart difficulties, and had bypass surgery. Sometime after the closing of the Foundation, he came to visit a colleague and me in our business office. He looked terrible, despite being his old, cheerful self. He had lost an enormous amount of weight, and his face was blue with lack of oxygen. He admitted that he was on his last legs, and wondered if there was any way that we could provide him with an experience before his departure. It had been a number of years since he had had one, and he wished to reacquaint himself with the levels he hoped to enter.

We promised to give it some thought. After he left my colleague said to me, "Certainly we have to honor his request. We now have MDMA, and it is such a remarkable material, what a wonderful way for us all to pay our last respects."

I could feel fear grip me. "Yes, but MDMA is a pretty powerful stimulant. The major contraindication is with heart patients. We could end up with a body on our hands."

"So what?" said my friend. "He's just about dead anyway. He could die at any time. If he dies, no one would be surprised. What a marvelous gift for him. I'll be glad to take responsibility for him."

I agreed it would be a marvelous gift, and deeply admired my friend for facing the situation and being willing to carry it out. I inhaled deeply, and pulled myself into the space of agreement and willingness to see the project through.

Several of us were present and joined Jeffrey in taking MDMA at the 120 m.g. level. I thought Jeffrey looked tense and worried. However, as the effects came on he went outside and became absorbed in studying plants and flowers. His concerns dropped away.

We took a 40 m.g. supplement at the 1-1/2 hour point. As we relaxed indoors, all the lines disappeared from Jeffrey's face, and he became very young and very alive. The earlier pallor completely left him. Jeffrey radiated warmth, and began to speak eloquently of the wonder, goodness, and beauty that pervades the universe, and the enormous gratitude he felt to the Supreme Maker of it all. He pointed out how everything created had its appropriate place, and how wonderful it was to peacefully flow with the Life Force in all of its seasons. His talking lifted us all into appreciation of these levels of awareness. My colleague later joined me in the evaluation that this was our most spiritually realized experience yet with MDMA.

Jeffrey was rejuvenated by this experience. His color came back and he was filled with enthusiasm. For several months he had been inactive. Now he resumed some former projects, including working with elderly people. He continued this activity for another six months before he once again became infirm. We discussed another experience, but he knew his time was up and that he might not endure it. He was very grateful for the additional six months of active life that the MDMA had given him. Even more so, he was content with the perspective he had gained on his life, and was ready to move on.

### *Jules*

In the course of a lifetime one meets a great variety of people. It is the outstanding ones that capture our attention. Jules is certainly one of those. Dynamic, full of life, bursting with humor, a skilled therapist, he was deeply committed spiritually. This commitment was the central core of his life.

Jules was even more outstanding in death. At the age of 33, he contracted cancer and fought a successful battle to complete remission. This experience gave him the understanding to be of profound help to others suffering from cancer, and aid them in conquering this enemy.

Thirteen years later Jules underwent bypass surgery. He lay in intensive care hovering between life and death. At times he seemed on the path to recovery, only to have this followed by a relapse. Sinking low, expecting the worst, he rallied again and again to extend his battle. This continued for seven painful months. At last, after a final surgery, internal bleeding brought him to the end. But not before he awoke sufficiently to cheerfully say good-bye to his family and close friends.

Jean and I recently attended a memorial service for Jules in his back yard. Over fifty people gathered there to give testimonials and pay their last respects. We had never witnessed such an outpouring of love and appreciation. It included the intimate sharing of family members, statements from close, dear friends who deeply appreciated Jules in his various personality roles, descriptions of the support Jules had given to neighbors in difficulty, and most impressively, reports of clients who felt their lives were given to them by Jules's ability to help them climb out of deep holes into the daylight.

All of Jules's close friends had rooted for him and prayed fervently as he lay helpless in intensive care. During this excruciating vigil, we all had a chance to confront death and what was happening with Jules.

At first we understood his eagerness to cure his illnesses and come back to life. But as he wasted away physically to the point where it seemed there were few resources to bring back, and as medical bills mounted astronomically, we wondered in different ways. What was causing the recurring relapses after each indication of gain? Practically all of us believed in reincarnation, and knew the faith Jules had in the survival of bodily death. Was he afraid to go on? Each in our own way pondered death and its meaning.

The full impact of Jule's message for me personally hit me in a morning meditation. There are many approaches to spiritual development. One broad class involves total surrender to God, being completely in the moment, and going with the flow of life. Another approach, perhaps best exemplified by Michael Murphy in his book *The Future of the Body*,[3] involves recognizing our unlimited potential and doing what we can to realize it. Jules firmly believes in this latter approach, as do I. It involves applying ourselves as best we can to develop the skills, perception, wisdom, and love to function at ever higher levels.

This latter method provides the ability, I believe, to generate ever more power, to be an ever-increasing force in the world. Yet it is a dangerous path, as the ego loves power. The challenge is to keep an appropriate balance.

The solution for me lies in the concept of partnership with God. It is this partnership which we each must individually resolve. If we rely completely on God to carry out our functions, nothing tangible will happen. On the other hand, if we try to do it all ourselves, we become warped, distorted, cut off from others, and do not have the vital energy or perception for appropriate actions. By being in tune with God, the power of the universe is with us. I can give a great deal of personal testimony as to the futility and drain in personal vitality that comes from thinking I can do it alone.

Jules was on the brink of developing immense power. For seven months he lay as a true warrior, facing incredible pain and anguish as he rallied his personal resources to heal his body. But in the end, it was not enough.

Watching Jules, I clearly see the importance of being totally open to all sources of help. Yes, it is my responsibility to set the direction. But only by surrendering to the situation, being completely open to all the forms of help available in the universe – the strength of friends, the love and compassion of the wise sages that have preceded us, to that remarkable healing energy that comes through the Grace of God – can powerful obstacles be overcome. I felt it a true warning to me to be careful of my striving, to avoid attacking barriers by brute force and severely taxing my personal resources. I must remain open and relaxed, be available to all the resources that exist, and allow them to nurture and support me. In this way I can truly achieve my potential.

Thank you, Jules, for your brave example, for your true spirit, and for the inspiration you brought to us all.

### *Edgar*

Spending a few days with our good friend Edgar has given me much to think about concerning the use of the sacraments.

Edgar and his wife Grace are among our oldest friends. We first became acquainted in the Sequoia Seminar, which initiated our spiritual search. They were among the first to go through our program at the Foundation, and were enthusiastic supporters of our work. They both felt that they had received a great deal of benefit from their experiences, and had opened up to many new possibilities in life. They found much personal understanding, a new sense of peace and fulfillment, had considerably improved their marriage relationship and communication with their children, and had opened up appreciably to spiritual development. This last they considered to be the most important of all.

Because of their character and experience, they were often chosen as "sitters" to take people home and be with them after they had undergone a psychedelic experience at our Foundation. When it became apparent that persons who had gone through the Foundation program could benefit from meeting and discussing their experiences with others, Edgar and Grace formed and led a group for this purpose.

They have both been willing subjects in our exploration of new compounds. They have continued to reap benefits, and have often told us how much they are indebted to us for making these experiences possible.

Edgar is a remarkable human being. He is a large man, powerful and strong, yet under the right circumstances he is like a warm puppy-dog. Edgar has amazing endurance, perseverance, and exceptional energy. He drives himself hard, and his body shows the signs of strain. Once he has adopted a goal, he latches on like a fierce bulldog, and cannot be deterred from proceeding full-bore until it is completed.

He loves to be in control. Edgar has remarkable confidence in his own ability, which is quite considerable, and can sometimes be quite stubborn. He is blessed with a saintly wife. Grace has been extremely supportive, and has grown considerably as she has handled difficult situations.

Edgar is extremely talented. He is very bright, and an outstanding inventor with good management ability. For years he was intrigued with the process of creativity. Working jointly with a good friend also interested in the creative process and in the mechanisms of the human mind, they came up with some practical, working rules to foster the creative process.

Edgar was fortunate to accumulate some capital through successful investments. At age fifty-five, he had enough capital to retire. But he was restless, and eager to place his knowledge of creativity to work in a successful business. He found MDMA to be an excellent tool to enhance his creativity.

But here we see manifested one of the real dangers of psychedelics. Unless used with wisdom and the kind of objectivity that comes from a good peer group, their use can powerfully reinforce one's strongly held views. In the case of his first independent endeavor, Edgar's single-minded approach, great confidence in his superior intelligence, and unwillingness to listen to advice from others led to substantial financial losses.

Humbled and wiser, he set out on a new project with equal determination but a great deal more care. This project was a very insightful one, and in addition involved genuine service to the market he envisioned. It was a herculean task; it involved gathering an enormous amount of essential information that would be of use to designers everywhere. The success of the work would depend on how completely all of the basic information was covered, how interestingly it could be presented, and how quickly specific information could be found.

When the time came to approach publishers, he found immediate response. Edgar ended up with a very favorable contract, and at the time of our last visit with him, had only four months more work to complete the project and send it off to the publishers in camera-ready form.

As we visit with our good friends, Edgar and his wife, we tacitly agree to spend a day in communion with the sacraments. The choice is the one which Jean and I have found to be so effective, 2C-E.

As we get into the experience Edgar becomes quite uncomfortable, and has heavy, disturbing feelings in his body. I have several suggestions to offer as to how he can ease this discomfort. This involves his willingness to let go and allow the inner feelings to surface. However, Edgar refuses any suggestions. He is so heavily defended against these inner feelings that he denies that his discomfort has anything to do with any inappropriate behavior or attitudes. When it becomes quite clear that he wishes no help and does not wish to deal with his feelings, we leave him to himself and pursue our own experiences.

The next evening as we are reviewing our journey together, Edgar shares that he experienced that everything is perfectly fine just the way it is. Yet in further discussion, he is quite aggressive and judgmental of others. As I wonder out loud if he considers his position "perfectly fine", he asks if there is any problem between the two of us. I reflect carefully and say, "No. But I do feel very sad that you suffer so physically and don't want to find ways to ease your pain".

This greatly irritates him, and he attacks me for thinking I can solve his problems. I get defensive and complain of his lack of trust in me and the fact that I might have learned through the years some useful approaches for resolving difficulties.

Not feeling any real heat, and realizing the investment Edgar has in his position, I said, "You win, Edgar", and we went to bed amiably. But on waking up the next morning, I thought deeply about it.

Is there any benefit from subjecting Edgar to a psychedelic experience when he is so completely resistant to making use of the opportunity? After all, he is deeply engrossed in an extremely important and valuable project, is under great pressure, and needs every ounce of his resources to fulfill his contract with the publisher. I provided him a day of discomfort and possibly introduced a whole new spectrum of concerns to preoccupy him, just when he most needed his resources to complete his work.

Of course I wouldn't knowingly do this. I certainly have some basis for considering that such an experience would be helpful to him.

I would like to use this occasion of sharing an exploration with Edgar as a basis for presenting some of my hypotheses about the nature of these experiences. These hypotheses are an intuitive integration resulting from participating in and observing a great many experiences.

I must first say that to my knowledge, from discussing the chemical action of psychedelics in the body with some of the most informed people that I know, that despite much speculation, there is no agreed upon understanding of what is actually taking place in the body to achieve the remarkable results observed.

When a person ingests a psychedelic, there is an enormously complex set of variables: the person's psyche, which includes his value-belief system, his life experience and conditioning; the state of his body; the environment he is in; his preparation for the experience; and the action of the chemical itself on these various factors.

The most important action of the chemical is to dissolve the barrier between the conscious and unconscious mind. This potentially provides access to all our forgotten memories, repressed feelings, hidden motives, drives, values, and habits as recognized by Freud. In addition, the unconscious includes the various dynamics proposed by Carl G. Jung. These include the archetypes of human behavior in all of its forms, and the Collective Unconscious. These are elaborated upon in Appendix IV, where I describe my view of the nature of the self and realizing our true nature.

But I believe there is something else that is quite important. This is the relationship between the psyche and the body. Alexander Lowen, in his book *Bioenergetics*,[4] sets forth this relationship between the psyche and the body, and the flow of energy. He describes how psychological characteristics produce physical armor, and affect body structure and movement. Thus correlates of our psychological dynamics appear physically in our body.

I am personally convinced that neurotic patterns have corresponding stresses and toxins embedded in our musculature, which result in the dynamics postulated by bioenergetics.

This means that even when one becomes aware of one's psychological problems, the toxins and armor are still stored in the body. Psychosomatic medicine takes a lot of this into account, indicating that disturbances like ulcers, heart disease, colitis, etc. have psychological foundations. Even after psychological insight has been gained, these toxins are much harder to remove, and yield only with the continued application of effort to free oneself of one's psychological problems by changing one's behavior.

One of the properties of a good psychedelic, which I believe is not well known, much less understood, is that *it can clear the body of toxins and armor that accompany the psychological dynamics.* Muscle tensions and stresses are relieved, so that the bioenergy that Lowen discusses can flow more freely, with accompanying improvement in mental-body balance. Consequently at the end of a good psychedelic session, one has a sense of bodily renewal and freedom (if it has been a hard-working session with a lot of repressed material released, it is not unusual to feel tired afterward. Consequently it may take several days to feel the full effects of such rejuvenation). Behavior is much easier to change when the body is free of this load.

This opening will last for a while, but can be dissipated if one continues in one's old behavior patterns and thereby rebuilds the toxins and the armor. Probably a great source of disappointment for a large number of people who ingested psychedelics in the 1960s is that because of the power of what they learned, they expected the experience to change them. Consequently they did not put in the effort required to change. The resulting discomfort of returning old patterns of behavior was often countered by a subsequent experience. While a certain amount of change inevitably takes place, the presence of continuing uncomfortable symptoms can lead to disillusionment, or new defense patterns to hide the disappointment. For the person who genuinely wishes to change, the window of opportunity following a good psychedelic experience is an advantageous time.

So now back to Edgar. For complete rejuvenation, the psychedelics, or as I prefer to call them, the sacraments, work best by ingesting them and being willing to focus one's complete attention on the experience that results. By holding one's attention on feelings that surface, the feelings eventually resolve themselves, often with an enormous breakthrough of understanding and release of repressed energy. It often helps to stay focused on the feelings by consciously breathing through them.

But suppose that one doesn't want to examine the feelings? They can be quite uncomfortable. Or the resulting insights can so oppose dearly held beliefs and actions that discovering the true nature of one's uncomfortable feelings would be terribly painful. In such cases one might well want to avoid them completely.

As long as the individual is reasonably honest and cooperative, there is still some benefit just from the release of the toxic material and the armor. Tensions can be relieved and new energy sources can be tapped, at least temporarily. And it is always possible that with the passage of time, a person may review what has happened and be more willing to allow feelings to surface at a comfortable pace. For it has been my experience (and more so lately as I have become more observant) that crusts are dissolved from the defensive walls that have locked down repressed material. This, along with any new learning that may have taken place during the journey, can permit such material to come to the surface more freely in the days following such an experience.

So it is possible that there can be gains for a participant even though he or she is not particularly willing to deal with unconscious material that is loosened during the psychedelic experience. And of course beyond what we consciously observe, there is a significant amount that transpires at various levels of the psyche that can lead to improved functioning with or without our conscious cooperation.

With these reflections on our experience with Edgar, I did not feel that I had done him a disservice. Fortunately, this was confirmed about a week later in a phone call when he reported that he had gotten considerable rejuvenation and renewed inspiration from our time together.[5]

### Chapter 10 Notes


1. Grof, Stanislav. *LSD Psychotherapy.* Pomona, Calif: Hunter House, 1980.
2. Meduna, L. J. *Carbon Dioxide Therapy.* Springfield, Ill: Charles C. Thomas, 1950. See Chapter 1, note 4.
3. Murphy, Michael. *The Future of the Body.* Los Angeles: Jeremy P. Tarcher, Inc., 1992.
4. Lowen, Alexander, M. D. *Bioenergetics.* New York: Coward, McCann, & Geoghegan, 1975.

5. Another explanation of the bodily rejuvenation that comes from a good psychedelic experience can be drawn from the practice of meditation. Psychedelics can so increase the intensity of the inner light at the core of our being that this light dissipates the toxins. Often in a good meditation session, stiffness, soreness, tiredness, and arthritic symptoms are relieved.

# Chapter 11
# Good Friends Along the Way II

## *Gil*

Gil is one of the closest friends I have. We met in the early 1960's, when Al Hubbard was attempting to enlist the backing of the Compudyne Corporation to support his enterprises. Gil was one of Compudyne's bright young men, who instantly formed an immediate rapport with Hubbard. He proved to be a very skillful traveler on the Hubbard space flights, which led to a deep friendship between the two. It wasn't long until Gil became a major supporter of Hubbard's work.

Financially, Gil and I were the two major contributors to Hubbard Enterprises. There was a major difference. Hubbard hoodwinked me out of every contribution. My gifts were described by Al as loans that would advance the cause of psychedelic research throughout the world. I expected the full return of my money!!

Gil, on the other hand, was a great deal brighter than me, and saw right through Hubbard's shenanigans. He ended up advancing more funds than I did. However, in his case he knew what was happening, and knew that he would never see his money again. His support was truly genuine.

Gil used the substances very effectively for learning and honing his skills. The result was that he became an extremely effective manager. Enhancing his very considerable native skills, he readily learned to separate wishful thinking, misperceptions, and defensiveness from facts. He learned how to quickly penetrate to the heart of a problem and instill clear communication. He established a track record and reputation that will always put him in demand, especially for businesses experiencing difficulties that need rapid resolution.

A strange affinity existed between Gil and me. We rapidly became fast friends. He had a marvelous disposition, and was full of energy and wit. He had no pretenses whatsoever, and was completely accepting. This made it easy to share intimately on any subject. We always had good times together. The deep bond we felt for each other is what brotherhood should truly be.

As he rose up the corporate ladder, Gil became very preoccupied with managing his companies, so that we seldom saw each other. So I was very pleased when he decided to retire at an early age, and we could spend time together.

He never lost interest in the sacraments. Exploration into the dimensions of consciousness was very appealing, and he was a skilled traveler. He knew the territory well, and had transcended many of the briar patches where I was still inclined to get snarled. He was eager to learn of the new substances, and we had great times exploring them together.

I found Gil an ideal traveling companion. He readily moved into expanded consciousness, a vantage point from which he was a source of wisdom and penetrating perceptions. Because of our deep acceptance of each other, we easily reached a deep rapport which allowed communication to flow freely. Our minds harmonized well and supplemented each other, so that we could have creative discussions and find ready answers to most of the problems we tackled. The following extracts from a journey we shared with 2C-E will indicate some of the ways that this substance can be useful.

At the time of this particular journey, Gil was immersed in several heavy problems. He was functioning at as poor a level as I had ever seen. He was facing some very difficult decisions in the work-place, and there were a lot of pressures from his marriage.

Gil had gone out of retirement to rescue a failing company engaged in the area of business in which Gil was most experienced. The money was appealing, as well as the chance to escape some of the domestic frustrations. I suspect that the principal reason was that it was hard to retire and allow important, highly developed faculties lie fallow.

At any rate, he had done a magnificent job in turning the bleeding company profitable, and now greater demands were being put upon him. Recognizing his talents, corporate management hoped he would cure two other ailing companies in similar fields.

Gil had considered several alternatives, and was not sure which direction to go. If management accepted his proposal, it would tie him up for several years with an intense effort, and would take a lot of energy. Another major problem was with his wife Grace, and with satisfactorily working out their relationship. Without her committed support, he would be unable to carry out the first project. A number of things needed to be resolved in their relationship.

> We both take 15 m.g. of 2C-E. As it develops, we find it very intense. We very much feel the heavy load we are both carrying, and struggle for quite some time to work our way through.
>
> Gil reports that this is the most uncomfortable experience he has ever had. He always manages to break through to the higher levels which are quite euphoric, and he has never mucked around in this kind of stuff before. We each proceed on our inner journey, working to resolve our troubled feelings. After two hours we feel that we have done enough at this level, and are ready to talk to each other.
>
> For the next couple of hours, we have extensive discussions about Gil's work situation. A lot of the problem stems from the Chairman of the Board of the parent company. He had backed the purchase of three companies to get their corporation into a new market area that looked appealing. They didn't know this business field, and paid too much for the companies. All three are taking formidable losses. The Chairman does not wish to acknowledge his error. He is hoping that Gil can put a program together to turn the companies profitable and rescue him, as he has done with the one company they hired him to manage.
>
> Gil is willing to do this, but he sees that it would be easier to scrap these three plants and start from scratch and build new plants. It would actually cost less money. But it might cost more than they are willing to spend.
>
> We spend a lot of time talking about his relationship with Grace and a lot of the difficulties he has in his marriage. Many of these difficulties are parallel

to those in my relationship with Jean. As we talk, I become much clearer on many of the aspects of my own marriage. I definitely see that one of the things that is holding back deepening the bonding between Jean and me is the lack of a complete commitment. There are times when I still like to sit on the fence and fantasize other possibilities. I see that if I cut out these escape mechanisms and focus the energy into our relationship, I could improve it considerably. As I share this with Gil, he sees that the same thing applies to his situation.

We share openly and deeply about many aspects of our life and our functioning. The exchange is fascinating, because we have quite different ways of evaluating data in many areas. Our enhanced perception causes each of us to examine carefully something the other sees of value that otherwise we might rapidly reject. We are both learning a lot from each other because of our different approaches.

Gil has always been very sure about what he wants to do. He's always felt that as soon as he became clear on his goal, then the universe cooperated to help it materialize. He has never been unsure of the right course of action. This was the first time in his life that he has been confused and really didn't know which way to turn. Gil usually gets the answers right away, and they are very clear-cut. This time they wouldn't come, and he got the message, "You don't want this answer".

As we talk we both feel much better. It seems very important to talk and share at the customary level. It also generates more data to work with when we withdraw inwardly to search our way to more comprehensive understanding.

I have been so deeply involved in my feelings that I am out of touch with Gil, and it is very difficult to get my head to work. Gil has a great need to talk about his business situation and his role in it, but I have a hard time following him. Usually one of the things I have greatly enjoyed during experiences with Gil is that we get into very clear spaces and we think very well together. We stimulate each other repeatedly to clarify the thinking of both of us.

Now I feel so sluggish that I have a hard time comprehending everything that is going on. I begin to see a number of very significant things. First, I see how my spending time to myself and being alone a lot of the time has focused my energy into a very narrow pattern of simply enjoying my environment. This has cut me off from communication to the extent that it is much more difficult to follow the affairs of the world. I see that I need to stay in better contact with others and their worlds and to listen carefully so that I don't withdraw into a rut.

The discussions with Gil are touching on many important aspects of my life. I see the investment I have made in psychedelics being a cure for the world. I want people who use them effectively like Gil to be outstanding in their performance and functioning. It is very important to me that Gil be very successful in whatever he is doing, because this would reflect credit on our path of using psychedelics. I also see how much I live vicariously through Gil, depending a lot on him and his abilities to make interesting things happen in my life.

I am constantly aware of the enormous turmoil involved in all of the issues that Gil has brought up as well as my own issues. Some of the things I ponder are like these: If the use of these substances makes one a more responsible human being and more capable of doing something worthwhile in the world, is Gil's management of a munitions supplying firm making a worthwhile contribution? Shouldn't it be possible for a person of Gil's very extensive skills and competence to make a much greater contribution to the world? And is this any of my business? How should the effect on other people's lives influence business decisions? For example, if Gil drops out, the company he has rescued may fail and the people in it lose their jobs.

On the domestic side, what about the rift between Grace and Gil as Gil continues to use these substances for greater understanding and Grace is reluctant to look into them? What about my own contributions? I have always hoped that Gil and I might do something together, but now I see I was relying on his skills. I need to develop something based on my own skills. Right now I feel a heavy resistance to my main project, which is evaluating and summarizing my work.

As time goes on and we thrash through all these different issues, a form of assimilation and integration gradually takes place. It is interesting how bringing all the issues into awareness results in improved well-being, even if the issues are not completely resolved. It is as though the inner computer is satisfied when it gets all the information. It can then work on this at its leisure. It is the withholding of information that is the source of discomfort.

The result is that we feel better and better. My mind clears and I am able to focus more completely on Gil's business problems and make some intelligent observations. My major contribution is to help him understand that his successful performance should be appreciated, not exploited. It is important for him to allow time and spaces for rejuvenation, or his skills and energy will be drained. And it is important that management recognizes this.

At one point he feels that he has a major breakthrough, seeing clearly the route that he should take in his business career. It involves being honest with himself and with the situation; the other people can accept the consequences or not, he doesn't really care. If they accept, fine, he will carry out the project. If not, he feels that he has already made a major contribution with which he is satisfied, and he can leave with a clear conscience. He also becomes quite clear about what he wishes to resolve with Grace.

I notice that when talking to Gil, it pulls me out of some of the turmoil of my feelings into another level of functioning. I call this level consensus reality. It is a good place and has a good feeling, and is a position of objectivity over one's thoughts and feelings. I am confident this is the level on which we eventually want to come out, in tune with our fellow beings. It is at this level that feelings of love and warmth build up, a stabilizing, comfortable level. It is no doubt at this level that therapy works. There seems to be something much more satisfying about it than just being with your own thoughts in your own head.

One of the things that has puzzled me through the day, especially the early part of the day, is that I have not been able to feel close to Gil. In the past I have always felt great around him, and we've always had good times in these experiences. Now I feel no warmth for him at all, and in fact I am inclined to look at him very coldly and with great detachment. However, I find this is true with me right now with everyone in general, so that I feel that I am working through my own very deep coldness and aloofness. As the day wears on this dissolves steadily, and I begin to feel closer to Gil. By the latter part of the afternoon, I have moved into a place of euphoria.

This is helped significantly by a further withdrawal with music. I put on Gounod's St. Cecilia Mass, and it is exceptionally beautiful. It lifts us both into a different level of experience. I feel God right before me, and feel that I can communicate with Him. Before, I felt that to follow the Fenelon prayer[1] I simply made myself as open as possible and flowed with whatever happened. Now I feel that I can ask for specific outcomes.

I ask what is the most important thing for me to learn. The answer comes back with great certainty, Love is the only answer. I experience loving in many aspects and many dimensions, and it is gloriously rapturous. I then ask why I have to suffer so. The answer comes to me that I was not present during the agonizing part of the experience. In other words, the heart of this experience is the opportunity to communicate with God. I was simply laying back and letting happen and didn't have any feeling of being in God's Presence. I remember the part of the prayer that says "I present myself to Thee" and I had not really presented myself. I was just laying there and letting things happen.

So now I present myself. I have the feeling of looking God straight in the eye. This is very, very difficult, and requires gathering up all of my being, all my strength, and all of my determination, just focusing directly ahead of me. This is a wonderful experience, and the skies open up and I see all the profound beauty in the clouds, in the mountains, in my surroundings. The sluggish feelings that I have been experiencing dissolve.

I see that I can heal my uncomfortable feelings by pouring love into them. And yet I have to do it carefully, because I don't want to get into my old error of contriving these situations; I want it to come from the Source. I see again that I need but to focus my attention in a given direction and allow God or the Universe or my deeper Self, whatever you want to call it, to simply carry out the action and fulfill the reality. This is a wonderful, magnificent feeling that glows throughout my being. The euphoria grows along with the deep feeling of love and well-being and warmth within myself.

It is getting close to sunset and we walk out on the land to my favorite flat rock. Now I am feeling an intense closeness with Gil, and it seems that the two of us together are generating an immense energy field. Even Spatzy, our oldest dog, now crippled with arthritis and who has not been more than a hundred feet from the house for the last two weeks, has walked over to the rock with us. This is a distance of about two hundred yards. We enjoy the beauty of the setting sun and the vision around us with all of its colors and shadows and light. We walk back to the house very content.

We both feel that we have done an extraordinary amount of work. We have had an enormous struggle and have worked through the things that have bothered us, and have come to areas of resolution. I still feel quite tired and a bit of latent sluggishness, which is characteristic for me with 2C-E. I take this as an indication that I am not being totally and completely in the moment. I therefore welcome it as a helping signal.

The next day is remarkably different. All the dregs of the experience, which the 2C-E so effectively allows into consciousness, have totally disappeared. I feel extremely energized, along with a very deep and satisfying euphoria.

Gil and I review the previous day as we talk together. It is very satisfying to be in his presence. He is enormously grateful for the experience and for the opportunity to come through all the confusion and once more reach clarity. He feels that a great, great deal had been accomplished. He leaves early, as he is anxious to talk to Grace and reach some agreements with her. He will then prepare for meeting with his company the next day and getting his business plans on track.

I find 2C-E is a remarkable working material. I discovery it makes me go deeper into my unnecessary garbage and keeps me at it until it is resolved.

The following day I feel a great deal freer and that things have been done at a very deep level.

The wonderful freeing of the foregoing experience was followed by a setback in which some of the old, uncomfortable feelings returned. I began to recognize a pattern. The experience dissolved some of the powerful walls of resistance holding down deep layers of repressed material. With these barriers weakened, such deeply buried material can work its way to the surface in the days following the session. I have experienced a day or two of this following each significant exploration in the last year or so, and am now becoming more aware of it.

Following the uncomfortable eruption, I settle into a space of peace. This is helped by recognizing that new energy has been released and can be focused into the new areas of realization to help make them permanent.

This new space incorporates such features as the feeling of a newly cleansed being with space and emptiness within, the feeling of oneness with my surroundings with no intervening barrier, the ease of getting into deep meditation in a matter of minutes to drop tiredness or any other negative feeling, clarity of thought and perception, the ease and value of being completely in the moment. There is a profound realization of the impossibility of avoiding pain, and being much more aware of its presence. It seems that for me a requirement of reaching this stage of awareness has been the willingness to accept and experience pain.

A big puzzle still is why I have had to experience so much pain. I am sure my future learning will shed more light on this. For now, I can see this ground has been hard-won through the willingness to totally experience whatever has been presented for me to experience, no matter how painful, and the outcome has been worth it many times over.

## *Tim*

I met Tim quite by accident. His son was in custody of close friends of my son, who were all visiting us. Tim came by to pick up his boy. This proved to be an important door opening for Jean and me.

I took an immediate shine to Tim. We shared common interests, and it soon became clear that Tim was one of the courageous explorers who tenaciously held out for the highest realization. He exuded kindness, gentleness, and wisdom.

My son often had difficulty hiding the fact that he is one of the special persons who clearly understands the workings of the universe. I was most impressed with Tim's ability to be patient and gentle and see Jerry in the highest possible light.

Our interest was mutual, and we knew that we must see more of each other. This turned out to be difficult, and it wasn't until two years later that a sound opportunity evolved. I was baby-sitting my two granddaughters in Burbank so their parents could take a trip to Germany. Daytimes were free and I was able to catch up on previously missed opportunities.

Our meeting resembled soulmates coming together. A radiant energy came from Tim. As we each shared what was most meaningful to us, we nudged and inspired each other into a near-transcendental state of being. We were both excited by the other's work; we agreed to spend time together for mutual exploration.

Loving our part of the country, Tim came to see us first. The first morning we were together, Tim introduced us to some of his techniques. He asked us to lie on the floor and relax while he put on some intriguing music. We followed his instructions for breathing a little deeper and faster than normal without tensing up. As we did this, we were encouraged to allow our bodies to vibrate and shake. Much to our amazement, with his encouragement and judicious placing of his hands on tense parts of our body, we both began to shake with considerable frenzy. We worked off a surprising amount of repressed energy that had been locked in our bodies by literally shaking it out. It took a little over an hour, and left us feeling greatly relieved and refreshed. This was followed by a stimulating hike in the grandeur of the High Sierras.

The following day we explored together with 2-CE, which was new to Tim. He had been excited about my personal reports and was anxious to try it. The following is the account of our journey:

> We all take 10 m.g. each of 2C-E. Following Tim's suggestion, the day is directed to an inner journey. It is very rewarding to sit in a chair and focus inward, following inner feelings. After the first hour the going gets sludgy, as is often the case with me using this substance. Staying focused on the feelings works off repressed material, but the feelings seem to continue to grow more powerful and more uncomfortable. Tim's advice is to stay with it; in time the feelings will be resolved. This confirms my previous experience, but I wish I could find a more pleasant way to do it. However, Tim's advice increases my determination to focus more directly on the inward process.
>
> About three hours later, Tim and I each take 5 m.g. more 2C-E. I continue the same process as before. At first events go much more rapidly; I threaten to explode into some new, expanded level. But then I bog down again, sinking deeper and deeper into what feels like a wall of totally solid hatred and resentment. In the past I have always used my head to find some approach to get out of the discomfort, like focusing on love. This time I was determined not to use any volition whatever, and simply see where the experience took me. This is extraordinarily hard work, and takes much determination and persistence. Yet I am determined to find the outcome of this approach. I hope I can drop these miserable feelings once and for all.
>
> I very much feel my irritation for certain specific people. Jean is one of them, as I find her attitude very caustic a great deal of the time. However, my resentment goes much deeper, until I feel I am occupying the general pool of hatred and suffering that permeates the world. I discover that I am in the middle of the general condition that currently pervades humankind on earth. I am desperately searching for resolution, realizing that what I am seeking for myself is also the answer for the whole world.
>
> Once in a while I take a much needed break to look outside and talk briefly with the others. We are all on our independent journeys, and don't wish to interrupt our work. I am completely concentrated on resolving the miserable inner feelings.

I begin to get some interesting insights accompanying my release of feelings. I see that a lot of my anger is caused by me not being myself, and not saying what I really think and feel because of my fear of what others will think. I see very clearly my constant catering to others, trying to please them. I spend a lot of time on this dynamic, but never feel that I reach the initial cause of this pattern.

At mid-afternoon I begin to feel somewhat better, and start getting more insights. One interesting sequence of events is looking at situations that have irritated me. I see that I was right to feel the way that I did, but that there is a better response which makes everything whole. An example is my irritation when Jean gets angry while I am describing the way something works. I see I am right, but need to find a better way to explain it to her. For a while I review one situation after another of a similar nature, with gratifying results.

I also see very clearly that the people I am irritated with are the ones to whom I don't express my true feelings. I hate myself for not being able to do so, but refuse to acknowledge my self-hatred and project it onto them. This went deep enough so that now, two days later, when I feel any irritation I look carefully at what's happening and see a satisfying resolution.

Tim is very much taken up by his own experience, and having a marvelous time. He greatly appreciates the compelling splendor of the surrounding rocks, desert plants and towering mountains. We are having a magnificent fall day. He is clearing up a lot within himself and enjoying it immensely. He is not interested in general conversation, but wants to hold it for later.

Jean is having a very beautiful day, very relaxed and enjoyable. She is quite content to be to herself.

I go off alone to my flat rock that I so much enjoy, and spend about an hour there. I feel wonderful being alone, engrossed in the exquisite countryside, now alive with light and energy. I am very much looking for answers, but again feel that I do not want to use any volition whatsoever, which is what I have so often done in the past. In fact at one point it appears that when I use pressure to create love or beauty, it is automatically followed by negative feelings, as this level of duality must stay in balance. The only way to find the peace I am searching for is to totally relinquish control and find the very Essence.

I realize that I am looking for a point at which I don't have to choose, where everything is blissful and taken care of perfectly. Yet at our ordinary level of functioning we exercise choice. This is all right, but we must be fully prepared to accept complete responsibility for our choice. I see myself making lots of choices, but unwilling to bear total responsibility for the consequences. This is generating a lot of pain. The consequences of many choices can be painful, but the pain is more bearable when incurred intentionally.

Back at the rock, I look up at the sky and am able to let go. I can feel various parts of my body relinquishing repressed energy. This feels marvelous. I want to know what truly exists if I let go completely, using no personal influence whatsoever. This is very frightening. Suppose there is nothing – no Supreme Creator in which to put one's trust!! I breathe through my fear and stay with it. At one point I feel I am on the edge of incredible, indescribable beauty that might be more than the body can stand. I do nothing to force it to develop, but simply wait and watch. I feel how marvelous is trust and patience. Everything becomes more and more clear, but it is surprisingly free of affect. I don't get into the euphoria and sense of inner well-being that I am accustomed to. But I stay with it for some time, as I feel I am clearing out whole areas of my body. The lack of joy doesn't matter, as I am dedicated to the search.

After a while euphoria begins to creep in somewhat, and I return to the house. My body feels extremely light and free; it is gratifying to simply observe everything around me while ceasing conceptual thought.

Tim has gone off to climb my meditation rock. Jean and I sit on the deck watching the sunset. The beauty is overpowering, and it is good to feel the warmth coming from another person. When the sun sinks behind the mountain, astonishing energy radiates up in the light rays glowing over the mountains. I have a great sense of the immensity we are immersed in, and though I am still somewhat blocked off from it, I feel very satisfied with my progress. I am steadily growing in the awareness of this enormity within my being. This is my goal and my intention.

All day I have not felt my usual sense of Presence, which I usually invite with volition. I make this invitation, and it is very fulfilling. I see that the way out of all the pain and suffering is in partnership with this Presence, feeling love. I know that only Divine love can heal the enormous rages I was experiencing. But I still have much to learn about how to avail myself of this love.

Three days later things are progressing well. The anger has dissipated, and I am very much at peace. I am taking it easy, letting things flow and insights appear without my usual compulsive searching. An ongoing awareness is building of the vastness of the inner light, and how without overtly pushing I can be an avenue for it. This inner light will ultimately clear up the discomfort I have so often carried with me. I can get a profound taste of this light by simply sitting and watching the clarity of the beauty that surrounds our home.

While this report may not seem much different than other experiences I have described, it is quite different in the naturalness with which it manifested itself. In no previous experience have I devoted the time so completely to the inner process. This is the procedure recommended by Tim. The result is that I feel much more work was done, and my whole being has freed up considerably. This has left a lasting improvement in well-being.

I have learned much about how helpful it is to breathe more deeply to relieve tensions that build up. This seems to provide more energy to allow the feelings to dissipate, while maintaining a relaxed state. At one point in the heavy part of this last experience, I could smell the repulsive odor of ether from a childhood operation for removal of adenoids. The fear associated with this operation has kept me breathing at a shallow level most of my life. I find that deep breathing creates more aliveness and brings more energy. This is no doubt another reason why I find climbing in the mountains so rejuvenating.

This experience cemented our relationship to Tim, and has laid the groundwork for continuing friendship.

## *Max*

I have commented on how experiences with psychedelic drugs are considerably enhanced with good companions. Should the friend also be a competent therapist, the enhancement is even more rewarding!

Max is a very good friend who has participated in a number of our research endeavors. Warm, personable, conscientious, he has made great personal progress over the last few years. He has been eager to investigate and train in various disciplines, constantly adding to his skills so that he may better serve his clients. Some of the skills embrace alternative treatment methods, such as using enhanced perception and bioenergy. These skills add significantly to his ability to heal.

We have enjoyed Max a great deal as a personal friend, and his increasing competence has served to add to the benefits that Jean, I, and other friends receive from our mutual explorations. The following are some illustrations of his ability to help, taken from our adventures together:

*Releasing feelings.* We take a walk, and in talking to Max, he makes some suggestions for dealing with the feelings I get caught up in. He feels that I stew in them instead of resolving them. Back in the living room, I work with him on this. He says it is important to say out loud what I am feeling. I do, moving into a feeling of utter tiredness and dejection. I say out loud, "It's too much". He asks me what is too much, and I suddenly realize that I am carrying the burden of trying to heal the whole world. I verbalize this, and he asks if I am willing to give the burden back. He says it is extremely important to consider each person in my life and give their load back to them.

This is an enormous relief, and brings overwhelming insights. I see with great clarity how I have assumed these burdens with my desire to be the healer, and how important it is to let every person be themself and do as they wish. These perceptions bring enormous relief. Then Max pipes up, "I'll bet you picked up a lot of it without even being asked!" With the penetration of this truth I broke down into uncontrollable laughter. What an outstanding release!

*Using energy.* Max and I are sitting in the hot tub. I report that I have a lot of pain and stiffness in my neck. He reaches over and puts his hand on my neck and asks me to relax. Very shortly I feel a warm, marvelous energy flowing into my neck, relieving the tension. Soon the ache and the stiffness are gone, and I have a nice glow within my body. What a superb talent he has!!

*Another situation.* Max is working with Elnora, who is having a very difficult time working through her feelings. I am enthralled by the skill he is exhibiting. I am completely aware of his kindness, his gentleness, his patience, his loving support, and his adroit questions which help to focus her attention on the issues that need resolving. My admiration for Max as a therapist jumps by quantum leaps as I observe him in action.

I see that in order to understand how to most effectively be of help, Max opens himself completely so that he deeply feels the excruciating pain Elnora is repressing. I gain still another profound level of appreciation for how a good therapist functions: I see Max's complete willingness to feel the depth of the client's pain so as to better understand it and work for resolution. I can feel it myself, and it takes great determination and detachment to experience that intensity of discomfort. Yet the depth of the pain is what elicits a corresponding deep compassion.

I express my admiration to Max for his skills, and appreciation for the depth of his supporting love.

He replies, "Thank you. But it doesn't do any good unless the other person is willing to let it in".

This comment drives home an important truth to me. All we can do is offer our help and support. It is still up to the person to decide whether or not to accept it.

### *Bill and Joanna*

At the beginning of Chapter 10, I described the special joy of sharing sacramental experiences with good friends, and the dynamics I think take place. But sometimes it is possible to experience bliss simply because of the very essential goodness of the other parties, and the high regard you hold for them.

This adventure with Bill and Joanna is such an instance. It illustrates how outstanding things can be when the conditions are just right. The conditions in this case include two exceptional friends, combining the wonderful qualities of great intelligence, being extremely competent, and who are warm, lovable persons. The other preeminent condition was a setting surrounded by nature in its full abundance.

We spent the better part of the day on the newly acquired property of our two friends. A magnificent house is under construction and much of it has been framed, with the floors of three stories already set in. We made ourselves comfortable in what will be the living room, looking through large open window frames over the surrounding grounds.

The front of the house is somewhat like the prow of a ship, so that there is a front window, about four feet high by six feet wide, and two identical windows on either side slanting back from the middle one, giving views in other directions. Beautifully designed, the house sits with grandeur on top of a hill, an ideal place of command over the surrounding countryside.

Out the windows, one sees a beautiful green meadow below with a good-sized pond off to the left. Patches of dark green give evidence of underground springs. The meadow is surrounded by a thick forest containing a great variety of trees. They are of all shapes and sizes, mostly conifers, but also some deciduous trees, blending tall, narrow forms with spreading branches. The entire area is covered by a variety of flowers, testimony to the sweeping proliferation and ingenuity of nature in providing an endless spectrum of patterns, shapes, and colors.

I find the most outstanding sight of all is looking through the central window directly at Mount Herman, a remarkably beautiful mountain in full view from the house. It rises majestically above the surrounding lowlands, to commanding, snow-covered heights. This readily becomes the focus of attention when peering out the windows.

Before leaving for the property, our friend Bill, Jean, and I each ingest 10 m.g. of what is proving to be our favorite sacrament, 2C-E. Bill's wife, Joanna, chooses not to imbibe. After the one-half hour drive, we are just beginning to feel it. We make ourselves comfortable in the living room-to-be, sit down to visit, and our experience develops rapidly. As my energy level rises, I can feel the enormous goodness of our host and hostess. Our combined energy sweeps me up to higher levels of realization, and I begin to experience penetrations of the Numinous. Despite my efforts at control, this brings forth considerable sobbing. At these moments the surrounding beauty is simply overpowering, and the sheer wonder of what I see completely takes me over.

When Bill and Joanna return from a walk, I immediately feel the wonderful energy coming from them, and once more approach an exalted state of consciousness. As I look at the mountain, the beauty becomes so intense it is hard to endure, yet it is so ecstatic it is worth totally surrendering myself to be at the complete call of whatever is orchestrating this experience. The joy of being in the presence of our friends is incredible, and I feel myself being carried into wonderful spaces. We are truly a remarkable group, and the 2C-E is an outstanding elixir. I keep repeating, the only way to describe this experience is that it is an enormous grace. Grace is what I continue to feel through and through.

As I sit looking at Jean, I search for her essence. I begin to feel a delightful, heavenly, exquisite love coming from her, that I consider the essence of femininity. It is very subtle, and I feel that I had erected numerous barriers to prevent it from reaching me. I allow the barriers to dissolve and the love grows in strength. This is as satisfying and wondrous a feeling as one can possibly want. I must, must keep this channel open. The feeling is so exquisite that it feels like the Divine Feminine Presence is at hand.

As I think about Bill, I see him as a noble soul – honest, just, and competent – one of the beings trying to bring integrity into the world. He has been fighting a hard battle with difficult forces so characteristic of many large corporations – the unconcern for the welfare of individuals, the demand for unquestioning obedience, irrational decisions made independent of those possessing the most intimate knowledge, poor communication, holding unjustified blame. It has greatly worn him down. Now he has chosen an ideal spot that is extremely nourishing. Here he can recover from the blows that have been dealt to him, gain strength and perspective, and once more be in a position to contribute.

This is a great paradox that I see again and again. The very sensitive souls are those with the capacity to discern and understand; they are in touch with their creative and caring levels. But because of their great sensitivity, they are the ones most hurt by the brutalities of the world. Yet this seems to me to be their goal in life: to gain strength so that they can handle the cruder aspects of life and still have available their sensitivity, so they can better serve the needs of the world.

Later I decide to join the others in a walk around the property. I gather myself up and focus all of my energy on being fully aware of my surroundings. When I walk out into the grasses and the flowers and the trees, I am simply overcome by the depth of the beauty surrounding me. Wherever I look is pure enchantment. Everything is glowing with God's magnificent presence. I yell at those ahead of me, "How can you rush so fast through such beauty?"

The high level of joy continues throughout the day, penetrating more and more deeply into my body. In the late afternoon Bill drives us down the

Jordan River, and again words cannot adequately describe the peace, the contentment, and the sheer beauty of the remarkable views. The river is an outstanding one, and lies in a broad, deep canyon composed of massive basalt cliffs, alive with color and intriguing surfaces. The banks are cultivated, revealing green fields and many species of trees, their branches waving in the breeze.

Everything that comes into view, even a freight car, seems charged with the glory of its own existence and full of significance. The all-pervading love binds everything together, and I can do nothing but simply open myself to the bliss and the wonder of it all. It is difficult indeed to muster sufficient gratitude to appreciate the inordinate beauty of this day, and the superb bliss of being in deep harmony with cherished friends.

## Chapter 11 Notes

1. The prayer of Fenelon outlines an excellent procedure to follow for a rewarding psychedelic experience. When I decided to take it seriously, it was a major factor in helping me achieve more beneficial experiences.

   It was recommended by the person whom I consider to be the outstanding psychedelic therapist on the planet. He claims to have personally introduced 3500 persons to a properly conducted psychedelic experience, as well as guiding 150 therapists.

   In the beginning he recommended a program of reading and study to prepare subjects for their first experience. In time he felt that the most effective preparation was to drop these suggestions, and simply ask the subject to read the Fenelon prayer aloud twice at the beginning of the experience. Here is the prayer:

   Lord, I know not what I ought to ask of thee;<br>
   Thou only knowest what I need;<br>
   Thou lovest me better than I know how to love myself.<br>
   O Father, give to Thy child that which he himself knows not how to ask.<br>
   I dare not ask either for crosses or for consolations;<br>
   I simply present myself before thee,<br>
   I open my heart to Thee.<br>
   Behold my needs which I know not myself;<br>
   see and do according to Thy tender mercy.<br>
   Smite, or heal; depress me or raise me up;<br>
   I adore all Thy purposes without knowing them;<br>
   I am silent; I offer myself in sacrifice;<br>
   I yield myself to Thee:<br>
   I would have no other desire than to accomplish Thy will.<br>
   Teach me to pray.<br>
   Pray Thyself in me.<br>
   AMEN. Francois de Salignac Fenelon

# Chapter 12
# Special Events

## *My Toughest Case*

Over one Labor Day weekend a number of years ago, my wife and I attended a three day conference at the Three Mountain Sanctuary.

The Three Mountain Foundation was founded by Richard Moss, M.D., and follows his principles of teaching. Richard Moss was once a practicing physician, but abandoned his practice when he discovered the value of the healing energies within us. Since that time he has devoted his efforts to discovering and teaching others how to get in touch with these energies and make them manifest in their lives. See Chapter 6, Note 5.

He has taught well, and we found this three day conference a powerful transformational experience. The staff has worked out group exercises and programs them in such a way that the group energy and level of love keep building to a climax on the last morning. I suspect that for many of the participants, they become aware of this level of energy for the first time in their lives.

And the same may be said for the level of love in the group. By the end of the conference, every member is practically in love with every other member of the group. Again, I doubt if they have ever experienced this level of love previously in their lives. So profound are the feelings that one cannot help but sense that the entire activity is divinely guided, and all of the exercises, practices, and activities are for the purpose of releasing divine energy into the world.

Out of the some twenty-five persons present, there was only one that I felt was a possible subject for our research, and with whom I cared to share the knowledge of our activities. His name was Jackson.

We broached the subject to him, and found him interested but frightened. We left it open for him to arrange for a visit to us if and when he desired.

We thought little more of it, so we were surprised a few days later when Jackson called and was rather desperate to come out. He was quite shaken up by the fact that Peggy, his live-in girlfriend of four years, had decided to abandon him. The reason was that Jackson had never been able to make up his mind sufficiently to make a commitment to her. She loved him and was a beautiful partner, but she had grown tired of his ambivalence and wanted out.

Jackson was quite stressed, which I didn't feel was the ideal state to participate in our research. After a few days he sounded better, and we agreed to see him.

Jackson proved to be a fascinating individual, and working with him turned out to be an extremely instructive involvement.

I had been drawn to Jackson because he was quite bright, articulate, and seemed deeply committed to his personal growth. I had overlooked many other factors, which began to become clear as we visited the day before our experiment. I had not given due credit to his fear, or to his pickiness. It turned out he had a variety of allergies, and was so fussy about his food that he had brought his own to the Three Mountain Conference. In the pre-day getting-acquainted talks, I began to see that he had constructed an amazingly effective system of self-defeat, which would turn every incident and development against himself.

Yet I had enormous faith in MDMA, having monitored a large number of experiences with no sign of any ill effect. So with my knight-in-white-armor attitude, we set forth to help rescue Jackson from his various dilemmas. What is that old adage about fools?

On the following day, Jackson takes 120 m.g. of MDMA. Jean takes 110 m.g., and I take 12 m.g. of 2C-T-2. This has become my favorite substance for accompanying others on the MDMA journey. It allows me to experience quite fully what the subject is going through, without the irritating effects that MDMA has on my prostate condition.

The ascent is nice, the energy rising pleasantly. We are in a good space in thirty minutes. Jackson feels the energy and responds well. We talk. At one point I happen to mention to Jackson that he isn't listening to me as I speak. This is the match that lights a bonfire. It starts by Jackson immediately losing his poise, and descending into the darkness of his bitter self-criticism.

He immediately embarks on the tale of his childhood woes. He is an extremely sensitive, delicate creature, and he was subjected to awful indignities by both his parents. He felt totally unloved, and manipulated purely for his parents' ends. He was constantly given orders for behavior, and his mother even had him wear a leash. His father was extremely authoritative, insisting on having his own way even if it took physical abuse. He hates both parents bitterly.

His younger brother by four years was not exempt from his ire, since the brother received what little attention the parents had to offer. Jackson is very much taken with getting as deeply as possible into his feelings, especially in the presence of two people devoted to careful listening. He brings up much anger.

At the hour-and-a-half point, Jean takes a 40 m.g. supplement of MDMA, Jackson 50 m.g. My dose of 2C-T-2 will last all day.

Jean is well centered, enjoying the experience. Jackson continues to get into his feelings. He has the most carefully constructed mechanisms of self-destruction I have ever witnessed. For example, he is starving for love. Yet he detests anyone who gives him affection, for they must be stupid indeed to love a miserable soul like himself. He refuses to do anything for anyone, because if they truly cared for him, they should do things for him with no expectation of return. In fact, the thought of doing anything for anyone else makes him extremely hostile.

What is there about a person which allows him to become so crippled? Were his family really that awful? Is he simply a remarkably sensitive person, crushed by the slightest fear of disapproval? Is there some enormous karmic burden that dictates that he must use every opportunity to punish himself until his inner debt is paid? These are great mysteries, but the bottom line is that Jackson isn't going to relinquish self-punishment without an enormous struggle.

Jackson is a very bright person, did very well in school, and passed the CPA exam with flying colors. But now he hates doing accountant work. With these proven skills, could he be so afraid of personal failure that he is frightened of assuming any personal responsibility? It is a remarkable dilemma, and promises an extremely busy day.

Jackson is determined to thoroughly examine his feelings, so Jean and I sit quietly by. At one point his rage is so enormous that I feel he can't properly discharge it except against some opposition. So I agree to pin him to the floor, and let him take out his anger against me. He is a small, slight person, and I am much bigger. Nevertheless, he has enormous strength, and becomes a mad, raving beast. It takes all of my strength to keep him pinned down. I am very glad that we have agreed to no violence, as occasionally when he slips out of my grip, he allows himself to be pinned down once more.

He discharges enormous anger in this way, but there seems to be no end to it. Yet he shows great courage and determination to get to the bottom of things. But I do notice that his attention span is only a few seconds.

So when he asks for a second supplement (I had mentioned the day before that other materials might be available), I suggest it might be best if he devoted the remainder of the day relating what he has learned so far to his life situation and the world around him.

But he claims that he is right on the verge of an important breakthrough. Ah, the perfect hook for me! How I would dearly love to seem him end the session with his feelings resolved, and ready to go back into life with new understanding and reserves! I had conveniently forgotten a situation twenty years earlier which had demonstrated how disturbed clients elicit your cooperation by this ruse of being on the edge of a breakthrough.

I agree a supplement might be useful; he immediately becomes frightened. We go back and forth on this for a while until I become convinced that he really wants to use more chemical, and I think it would do some good. So 5-1/2 hours into the session, he takes a supplement of 6 m.g. of 2C-T-2. I take the same to lighten the load I am feeling.

Jackson continues pretty much in the same vein, getting up much anger, at times appearing very beast-like. I give him a chance to role play with his parents, I taking the part of first one and then the other. This allows him to express more anger. I tell him that one day I hope that he can do this directly with them.

In the late afternoon we talk Jackson into taking a walk outside. He is reluctant, but accepts our suggestion. He finds it beautiful outside, and gets into some wonderful positive energy. However, he is quite weak and occasionally sinks to his knees. I feel it is his tendency to sink into inner experience. He has almost no faculty for taking command and making decisions or carrying out actions to overrule his feelings. He feels he is a bottomless, empty pit. I suggest that he fill it himself. He can concentrate on this only a short time.

I hope he will discover how desperately afraid he is to find out how much he acutely desires love. He shows little sign of this, so I begin to become more directive. I wonder if he felt helpless with his parents, and he looks at this. We discuss the importance of the rational mind, and the importance of being able to follow one's reason over emotions, the ability to act despite feeling fear, resentment, or other negative feelings. During the walk, we practice the ability to drop the inner workings of the mind and pay attention to what is around us. He succeeds somewhat and at times.

I share how important it was for me to learn gratitude and appreciation. He realizes that he never does. He is able to see the surrounding drama of the countryside, and appreciate it for a while. He acknowledges that it was good to go outside and experience the outdoors.

We discuss forgiveness. Back in the house, he goes inside himself and is able to forgive his mother, father and brother. There is much pain and realization, particularly with his brother. He recognizes his parents' limitations, and how he used his own unhappiness to create misery for his brother. He is beginning to see light at the end of the tunnel; he can experience some euphoria, good energy.

Feeling that he is much stronger and insightful, I mention that I see him as very consuming in his relationships, that it is no wonder Peggy is leaving him. He begins to get it. His initial response is to always feel hostile, as it is very difficult for him to take any advice or suggestion. I suggest he has to grow out of this and look at the reality of the situation: what is really going on? He needs to learn that everything is not an attack on him; he is the one who changes it to an attack. He should look at things on their merit. He requires complete retraining in this regard, as his patterns are so heavy and deeply set.

He has made much, much progress. I am on the sofa in the living room, and tell Jackson I am hungry, will he please bring me a bowl of soup. He says, "Get it yourself!"

I am flabbergasted. I say, "Good God! I have stood by you all day, answered your every wish, and now you can't even bring me a bowl of soup?!! I don't give a damn how you feel, I want some soup!!"

He gets it, and finds out it feels good to do so.

He wants to discuss his relationship with Peggy. I role play with him. He is still very torn. Now he understands how awful he has been; he discusses going back and serving her. Yet he still feels some repulsion in being with her. We discuss the possibilities – his fear of intimacy, his unwillingness to care enough to have to do something for someone, his fear of discovering his own self-hatred. We retire with this issue unresolved.

Jackson spends a sleepless night, and the next morning he is still unresolved about Peggy. He would like to go back and plead for her to stay with him; he will promise to change. But in his heart he still can't make the commitment.

I suggest he stay with us another day. We take a hike and do some good talking to integrate our experience. He comes to peace with the outdoors, and begins to feel much better.

Jackson showed an enormous amount of courage and persistence in facing his inner demons. The problem of now resolving them in his life will be the biggest task he has ever faced. The next few days will be the hardest. If he gets through them okay, I believe he will steadily gain strength.

Jackson returned home still ambivalent over his course of action. But this was settled by Peggy, who insisted on leaving. This was a hard blow for Jackson. Fortunately he had some friends and teachers whom he could rely on for support. But he had an agonizing time coming to terms with his experience and the blow of separating from his partner. He was in constant touch, and for a while was living on the edge. He gradually pulled himself together, and in time was able to return to a productive profession. He is now happily married and helping his new wife to raise her son.

## *My Most Rewarding Case*

Ralph is a very competent industrialist from New York. In his early sixties, he has accumulated substantial wealth through his creative designs and products produced by his company. He was visiting the Three Mountain Foundation, and upon hearing my name, wished to visit. He has had a long-standing interest in psychedelics, and has managed to share experiences with a number of the outstanding figures in this field.

We found him to be a very positive, energetic person, who much preferred talking to listening. He requested to participate in our research. I did not encourage him, for although he has had many outstanding experiences, there was little evidence of his incorporating his insights into his lifestyle.

But he was persistent and stayed in touch. He furnished evidence of important changes taking place in his life, and I was feeling guilty over my judgmental attitude and unwillingness to help when asked. So we set a date for an experiment.

In briefing him the evening before, I told him that he needn't bother with the tape recorder he always used. He continually carried with him tape recordings of previous sessions. These were recordings of beautiful, highly inspirational wisdom of the most profound sort. Many were the kind of aphorisms one might wish to supply to an aspiring seeker of enlightenment. Ralph obviously got much pleasure in playing these for people, and it was clear that part of his feeling of superiority rested on the outstanding perceptions revealed in these utterances.

Ralph was quite taken aback by my suggestion. I asked him if he would not prefer this time to concentrate on incorporating such truths into his lifestyle rather than just listening to the recordings. He agreed.

The next morning, Ralph takes 20 m.g. of 2C-T-2. Jean and I accompany him with 12 m.g. each. I stay light so that I do not get caught up in my own dynamics, and can be of maximum support.

As the experience develops, Ralph gets quite uncomfortable. He experiences a great deal of anger, which I encourage him to release. Later I look at him and see enormous fear in his eyes. I ask him if there is anything he is afraid of.

He replies that he is afraid of going crazy. I say, "All right. Go ahead and go crazy. Assume this living room is a padded cell. I will be the padding, and not let you do anything destructive, either to your self, anyone else, or anything in the room."

These words flowed spontaneously from me, and I knew I didn't dare to stop and think about the possible implications. Ralph is a good deal larger and heavier than me, and I might have my hands full. Yet I felt a strong inner confidence, and had no hesitation in proceeding.

Ralph begins to roar, emitting aggravating, bellowing sounds. He is pouring enormous feeling into his roaring. It takes a strong heart not to be frightened. He begins to gasp, and it looks as though he might throw up. Jean runs for a plastic bucket from our utility room and puts it in front of him. I encourage him to throw up in the bucket. He heaves and heaves, making deep, retching sounds, without expelling anything physical. After a few minutes of this the sounds diminish. Ralph seems spent and sits down to rest, looking out the window.

Ralph reports that an amazing thing is happening. As he looks out of the window, he hears his own heart beating.

Then he realizes that his heart is beating in synchronism with the central heart of the whole universe. The whole universe is beating together! Then he realizes that he and the universe are one, and he begins to sob. He is filled with joy, and the ecstatic feeling of being in harmony with all that is. He feels totally freed from all previous discomfort; he has achieved that most precious realization of which man is capable, the state of Union with All There Is.

Ralph is overjoyed. In spite of having had many outstanding experiences in the past, he had never before experienced this level of realization. He is filled with wonder and gratitude.

Simply being present to share this experience is very gratifying. There is a deep satisfaction in being open to inspiration, and knowing that things have worked out well.

I do not know how well Ralph has retained this experience, or how it has affected his day-to-day life. I do know, however, that it is an experience that cannot be forgotten. I cannot help but believe that in some way, even without conscious encouragement, the effect of such a contact with the Numinous creeps into our values and our thinking and our action.

There are places on the surface of the earth which people call "Power Points". The locations are invested with special significance, and it is claimed that they make available to earnest seekers aspects of Reality not ordinarily perceived.

I admit that there have been some special locations, like St. Paul's cathedral in Rome, and even some locations in nature, where I have sensed something special. These places have had an unusual impact on me. But in general I am afraid I am rather impervious to these energy fields and perhaps the ideas behind them, as exemplified by the fact that I feel nothing particularly special about the claimed vortexes in Sedona, Arizona. However, it is impossible to deny the impact of the outstanding beauty of the whole Sedona region.

If there are such things as power places, then Death Valley National Monument in California must certainly be one of them. And if it is, it must be because of the outstanding human events that have occurred there. Some of the foremost occurrences of my life have taken place at Death Valley. These have transpired while riding or driving through the valley under the influence of an outstanding sacrament. For this purpose, I know of none better than Sandoz's LSD.

If outstanding events, or powerful feelings, or being overcome with reverence, wonder, and beauty, can leave an aura like Sheldrake's description of morphogenetic fields,[1] then Death Valley is surely a power spot. I have had many such occurrences there, and I am inclined to believe that our continued profound experiences do build up such fields, as being in the valley is conducive to furthering such experiences.

This was driven home all too well in the following event. Our friend Max was visiting us, and when other invited guests failed to show up, it seemed an ideal time to introduce Max to one of our favorite journeys. It had been some while since Jean and I had conducted anyone on this tour. Years ago we used do it rather frequently. But we discovered that for a well-focused experience, it didn't make much difference where one was, and the comfort of our living room avoided many miles of driving. Yet for the candidate who is ready to take advantage of such an experience, the Death Valley tour is very difficult to beat.

And this was a very special occasion. We are very close to Max and have excellent rapport. And Max is a very eager and appreciative explorer.

We embarked on our journey, giving Max a full measure of what we deemed appropriate. Jean took one-half this much, and I took half again, agreeing to do the driving. I planned to take a like amount once reaching the valley floor, with the difficult part of the drive behind me.

There is always the question of whether the amounts chosen are adequate, considering such things as the aging of the substance and the possible psychic resistance of the imbiber. In twenty minutes I was feeling very little and beginning to get worried. Then Jean broke through and reported that she was quite intoxicated. Not too long after, Max was swept away, finding his dose as powerful as what he would ordinarily expect from three or four times the amount he ingested.

For myself, it was very slow coming on. By focusing on stillness and holding my mind quiet, it accentuated the progress of the chemical. I began to feel it more and more intently, and by the time we crossed the Panamint Valley, it was so intense that I wondered if I would supplement.

As we drove up toward Towne pass, moving into the remarkably colored mountains of the Panamint Range, the beauty grew greater and greater in intensity. There came into view an unusually sculpted, exposed section of mountain which my friends affectionately call "Myron's Grotto". It never fails to move me to tears. It is shaped like a huge grotto, with a pinkish-white, rough rock background. Carved out of the wall are many tall figures, in dark pinks and reds and whites, standing looking out over the Panamint Valley. To me they always appear as the guardians of Death Valley. They stand at the entrance inviting us in, and assuring our safe and worthwhile journey. They are the custodians of the higher regions, and as we pay them due respect, the treasures of the valley are revealed.

Now verbal descriptions become totally inadequate. Only the most artistic, articulate use of words can begin to convey the remarkable sights we behold. The mountain cliffs are saturated with color, and the formation of the gorges and weathering patterns unfold an endless variety of stunning visuals, each more beautiful than the previous. We are overwhelmed by the amazing variety of form, surface, and color. Somehow some deep hunger inside of us is assuaged by this massive variety of input, flooding us with beauty.

The beauty slackens as we reach the top of the pass, where we are surrounded by just ordinary grassy slopes. But descending the other side, the massive vista of the valley comes to view. Here is an amazingly broad expanse of flat surface, whitened by the remains of past floods of water. The water has long since evaporated, leaving behind the mineral deposits which mark its former presence. On either side of the valley rise mountain ranges with tumbling, distorted layers of sedimentary rock, in many places tilted by underlying igneous intrusions. The mountains are carved into a great number of narrow canyons, the result of endless eons of constant weathering. Everywhere is the same continuing variety of color, so that no matter where you look there is interest and beauty. And in the heart of the expanse of the valley floor are bare, wind-swept dunes of the finest, pure sand.

But the best is yet to come. Approaching the sand dunes, I take my supplement. Shortly after that we come to the area where the pupfish spawn. In the heat of the summer, when every trace of water evaporates, these remarkable little fish bury themselves in the mud and hibernate through the summer and winter. In the spring when water returns to the deepest sloughs, they come to life, bubble up, and swim into the water and spawn.

Jean and I had once visited here with two good friends to observe this phenomena. They were program writers for the company I then managed, Multi-Media Productions, Inc., a company that made sound filmstrips. The emerging of the pupfish was photographically recorded for a program they were producing. Viewing this area focused me on the company, and I sank into some miserable feelings. This was a very poor outcome, I thought, of taking the supplement.

But I remembered the various devices I have learned to get away from uncomfortable feelings. First I looked to see why memories of Multimedia made me uncomfortable. I saw many good things that had transpired, particularly the contributions of other people, that I had failed to acknowledge. I now did so, and this released my feelings. It was like unresolved karma that needed redemption. Now I could turn my attention to my surroundings.

Once more I focused on the stillness, held my mind steady, and began to appreciate the beauty of the valley floor. Like turning on a huge faucet, feelings of love and energy began to swell within me. As long as I stayed focused, these feelings rose to enormous proportions.

Now we turn south on the road that leads to the Artist's Drive. This part of the drive is particularly spectacular. The mountain range to the east descends until it extends into the valley in long, weathered mounds, almost like huge paws of giant animals kneeling, facing the valley. These hills are solid, fine dirt, deposited by the run-off from the higher elevations. Again the colors are remarkable, being all shades of chocolate and brown, with some light cream colors occasionally thrown in. The road is very close to the foot of these hills, and the intimacy makes them all the more spectacular.

At last we turn into Artist's Drive. We climb steadily to the very foot of the vertical cliffs overlooking the valley. Whatever I said before about colors, shapes, and beauty, is completely swamped by what we now face. It is absolutely indescribable. The colors are brilliant – fiery reds and pinks and greens and purples. But the textures – the textures are unbelievable. Surfaces full of holes of all shapes, thin sculptured layers of rock that look like veils, contours and shapes and surfaces never before seen, all alive with ever-changing color. In our state of clarity everything stands out in the most minute, remarkable detail. The beauty is overwhelming, and we are simply undone. We cannot look at such beauty without crying and crying. We are beside ourselves with joy and ecstasy. It seems that nothing on earth can equal the sights we are beholding, or match the deep stirrings of our souls that are taking place. We must summon enormous strength to be able to continue to watch it. The car moves slowly on, constantly revealing new surfaces, new colors, new vistas. It is almost more than one can take.

We crawl along for several miles, looking at one breathtaking view after another. And we are in the midst of it. You can almost reach out and touch some of the phenomenal formations. What magnificent artist assembled this astounding collection of visions? How did all of this beauty come to reside in this particular place? What greater evidence could one possibly wish for the astounding creator of our world? And how could one possibly express sufficient gratitude for this amazing experience we are privileged to undergo? Overwhelming, overwhelming, overwhelming.

We finally reach the Artist's Palette, and stop to pull ourselves together. We are still in the presence of an amazing variety of colors, and they are exhibited at this location in greater intensity and variation than anywhere else. Behind the remarkable display which is near the viewing point stand the tall mountains with their variety of formations and splashes of various hues. Beyond the Palette these huge cliffs provide an endless exhibition of wonders to be examined.

The drive continues through intimate hills and formations. Some look, as Max suggests, like Italian ices, with the flow of different flavorings poured over the mounds. Others have smooth, glassy, bubbly surfaces as though water were running down over them. And around some turns the high mountains in the background become visible, alive with colored patterns that according to Jean look like the designs on multi-colored Indian skirts.

At last we are at the end of Artist's Drive, and we return to the main road fully satiated. The sun is now getting low, and long shadows are creeping across the valley. But the surrounding mountain ranges take on new appearances in the soft, warm light of the setting sun. As we drive across the valley with the vistas spread before us, a new, soft glow overtakes them. This is the glow of our inner being, fully content, basking in the love of our mutual warmth, reflecting on all that appears before our eyes.

Throughout this astounding journey, I have numerous occasions to be grateful for various things I had learned in previous journeys. I am blessed to have a sense of the Presence, which as I pay attention to it, comes more intimately into awareness. I am grateful for my Tibetan Buddhist meditation training, which has helped me learn to hold my mind still, thereby offering the space for other dimensions of reality to present themselves. I am grateful for the ability to look with love and appreciation without manipulation, as only in this way can the more profound levels of energy, meaning, and radiant love reveal themselves. And as we depart the valley, once more passing the grotto, I become aware of the countless wise and enlightened ones who have gone before, and only wait to be asked to direct their love and support to enormously enhance our realization.

## *A Magic Journey*

I have described in the beginning of Chapter 10 the particular joy of journeying with special friends.

Two of our good friends are a remarkable pair. Edward is a kind, gentle, extremely sensitive soul who is practically a saint. He is deeply committed to the Divine, and lets very little stand in the way of his devotion. He is studious, well-read, and thoroughly grounded concerning the world's religions and spiritual literature.

His companion, Larry, is a totally different personality. He is a dear, gentle soul, – young, handsome, and warmhearted, a lovable comrade. Thoughtful, attentive, sensitive, he is always right there with support and assistance to anyone who may be experiencing discomfort. His own mind is very fluid so that he easily moves through different states of experience.

They live in a beautiful home in a wooded area at the foot of a commanding mountain. They have made their home an idyllic retreat for friends seeking respite from the tumult of modern civilization. Truly imbued with the spirit they strive to manifest, with discerning taste they have created a beautiful, restful, inspiring environment. Their garden is laid out tastefully with flowers in every nook, a beautifully designed mandala composed of brick laid in the soil, and plantings of trees and shrubs to provide a peaceful setting intimately in touch with nature. Restful vistas look over rocks, colored earth, and towering mountains in the background. The slightest breeze creates whispering among the branches in the surrounding trees.

Inside are tastefully selected furnishings, skillfully placed to provide for comfortable listening to music or for interpersonal discussion. Selected artifacts blend color and interest to provide archetypal connections to a higher state of awareness.

Best of all is the way each visitor is treated as a highly honored guest. Almost every need and wish is anticipated and fulfilled. Exquisite meals are provided with the same care and taste in preparation, so that each meal is gourmet.

I know of nowhere where one can be better treated than at the hands of these two caring, solicitous individuals.

Jean and I always look forward to a visit with our very good friends. Taking their spiritual dictum seriously, they always see us as manifestations of the Divine, and treat us accordingly. For persons like myself who are attempting to reach such a state of functioning, Edward and Larry are inspiring models. It is a great privilege to be on the receiving end of such genuine attention.

For our last visit they had a special treat in store for us. We piled into their van, which had been well prepared with food and supplies for our journey, and we took off for Canyon de Chelly. There Jean and I took a room in a comfortable motel. There was still enough daylight to drive around the rim of the canyon and examine some outstanding views.

I have seen many spectacular places on earth. In the past I rated first the Artist's Drive at Death Valley, viewed in the afternoon sun. Then came the Grand Canyon, and close on its heels the magnificent country surrounding Sedona. But all of those fade in ranking beside the grandeur of Canyon de Chelly.

The Canyon has a color close to the marvelous pinks of Sedona. But the high, sheer, massive cliffs, the sculpted walls, and the isolated towers of vertical rock depict a stateliness and might transcending that of any of the places I have seen.

The canyon walls are striking in every direction. Each turn reveals new faces, sculpting, and formations. Below the massive walls is a flat river bottom, covered with trees and cultivated fields. We are at the peak of fall, so that the trees are illuminated in brilliant fall colors – yellows and golds and pinks. It is pure magic to look over this inspiring landscape.

In the morning we hire a guide and walk down into the canyon. It is thrilling to step over the weathered, colored rock. At places we cannot see a path past the rapidly descending rocks, but our guide carefully picks the way. In some unusually steep locations, footsteps had been carved into the rock to allow safe passage.

At the bottom of the canyon, we can appreciate the high canyon walls in all of their magnificence. Simultaneously we walk past colorful cottonwood trees in their fall brilliance. The river bottom is dry, but the very fine sand and the numerous rocks strewn over the valley floor reveal their own display of the Supreme Artist's craft. The canyon floor is cool, but pools of sunshine offer opportunities to bask and throw off the chill.

As we walk, ever new faces, images, and massive sculptures come into view. Most anywhere on the canyon floor we are content to simply sit down and look. We could spend hours in any one spot examining the various surfaces of the cliffs, the structures and weathering patterns, the figures that can be elicited from the rocks. Overhead the sky is crystal blue, but with unusual wispy, curly clouds floating overhead that carry their own revelations of meaning. On many of the high ledges are the famous cliff dwellings where civilizations once resided.

Exposure to all this grandeur and beauty, in the presence of intimate friends, cannot help but unleash one's spirit to soaring heights. With this barrage of light and beauty, do we dare to enhance the energy with a sacrament? We do.

It isn't long before I begin to doubt the wisdom of this move. We were in a remarkable, loving state, bombarded with beauty. As I begin to feel my old initial discomfort on starting a sacramental journey, I wonder if I'm not being too greedy. This feeling intensifies as I become more and more uncomfortable.

A number of realizations come flooding in. My body is getting more uncomfortable, yet we had told our guide about ruins we wished to reach that were several miles away. I begin to think about the comfort of our living room, and how nice it is to be completely undisturbed and simply relax to the experience.

Then there is our Indian guide. A young man of around twenty-two, he is obviously moody and unhappy with life. When we had gone to the Visitor's Center that morning to select a guide, he was the only one who had gotten up early enough to show up. It was obvious that Edward relied a great deal on my judgment in making this important selection. At the time I saw nothing wrong with him, and approved his enterprise in being there early.

He no doubt is very sensitive, and begins to pick up my uncomfortable feelings. He is concerned with my age, and whether I can manage the steep descent, or for that matter the long walk. The more uncomfortable I become, the more unhappy he looks.

I find myself amazingly disturbed by the presence of our guide. I feel his unhappiness and judgment to the extent that it is spoiling my experience. Once more I deeply appreciate how in our work we have created a safe, comfortable environment, free of distractions, which allows the subject unrestrained experience. As my discomfort continues to grow, I too long for a situation where I can simply let go and be free.

My discomfort becomes excruciating. I yearn to collapse on the ground and allow my feelings to flow out and dissipate. I stop frequently to sit down and relax, and get some measure of release. This very much disturbs our guide, who worries about my physical condition. He obviously does not want the responsibility of over-taxing an elderly person. He gets more and more impatient as he sees that we are not going to make our destination.

Finally he says we must hurry, as he has an appointment to see a sick person in the hospital in the early afternoon.

At first I am even more uncomfortable, feeling the time pressure. Then I begin to wake up. I begin to realize how much I am allowing the guide to dictate my experience. Here we have driven hundreds of miles to take advantage of what Edward and Larry no doubt consider the greatest experience they can provide for anyone. Instead of appreciating the outstanding beauty and all that they have done to make this journey possible, I am fretting over pleasing our guide! I can feel Edward's deep disappointment in the miserable experience I am having, and in my concern with the attitude of our guide.

Feeling more myself, I speak to the guide. "When we hired you, you didn't mention any previous appointment. We don't care about any particular place to get to. We want to take our time. We've come a great distance to see this canyon, and we may want to take all day to enjoy it."

I speak in a firm tone of voice, and the guide immediately becomes contrite. He says that we may take as much time as we wish – all day if we like.

I feel very relieved with this settled. Both Edward and Larry are glad that I spoke up. From this point on I am more relaxed and begin to free up from the disturbing feelings. It is not long until the rewarding aspects of the experience begin to manifest, and I drop my uncomfortable feelings and turn my attention to the surrounding grandeur. Yet somehow the guide has deeply affected me, and I am aware of his distracting impact throughout the day.

Now a most marvelous transformation is taking place as the sacrament takes effect and all of my senses dramatically open up. This results in what must certainly be as much impact of light, beauty, and meaning that the human frame can stand. Each moment is absorbed in eternity. The wonder of the Supreme Artist overwhelms the conditioned mind. It is only by letting go of all preconceptions, values, dictates, that the mind can flow sufficiently free to begin to embrace the wonders being revealed.

All senses become wide open. It becomes apparent that everything in our surroundings can expand into new dimensions of detail, beauty, and clarity. From the minutest blade of grass to the huge walls of the canyon, I can observe a striking array of detail. The closer I look, the finer is the detail. I must surrender and open myself to allow this enormous expansion of input into consciousness. This results in a sublime feeling of release and exultation as I become increasingly in touch with new worlds of input.

To apprehend the worlds of new data, my own being must expand to encompass them. My individual self and its notions of personality are rapidly transcended to encompass the grandeur of the myriad dimensions of creation. What an exalted feeling!! How in the world can one find words to describe such a bombardment of overwhelming, exultant beauty?!! It is impossible to describe the privilege and the gratitude of being treated to such celestial glory.

At one point Edward and I confront each other. As we gaze at one another, I observe layer after layer of conditioning being stripped away until I am looking at the very radiant core of Edward's being! Again, words fail to describe the incandescent resplendence of this remarkable sight. We stop when we can no longer master the strength to hold steady before such splendor.

Later after climbing out of the canyon, we are back at our motel. We are sitting together on a little patio, looking out over comforting trees and lawns and up at a sky filled with wondrous clouds. The clouds are forming and reforming in magical patterns. We are reviewing the events of the day. As we sit and talk, the bonding among us deepens, and we feel utter contentment and gratitude.

I am drawn to the clouds. They always pull me out of myself and invite my participation; they promise rewarding excursions into new dimensions. I know I must be perfectly still. Fortunately I am able to do this. As I hold still explosions of energy take place, and images fly by. It settles down to stability, and in the stillness a new energy creeps into my being and fills it. Again I realize that it is in the stillness that God can become manifest. By being still, I provide an avenue for Him to enter the world and make His presence known. His presence is a burning fire of love. Holding still, I can allow this love to flow into the world and burn up the dross that encumbers mankind. How this is done and to what extent I do not know. I only know that this is the most wonderful and satisfying thing I can do, and brings me into exultation. In some mysterious way I cannot understand, I am confident that it opens a door somewhere for others to touch an exalted state.

This seems to me the best hope for the world. Ignorance, self-interest, and destruction are preceding at such rapid paces around the globe, there is no certainty that our civilization can be rescued. But if it can, it will most likely be by those who are willing to become channels for this Divine love and hold steady against the pain, suffering, and ignorance of mankind. If enough join this enterprise, then I am convinced that sufficient light can be brought to bear to eventually help people wake up.

I take a good look at Edward. During the day I had become aware of how he holds off a certain amount of glory by not considering himself worthy of accepting the full impact. As I look at him I see a beautiful, magnificent being, a true saint, totally committed to God's work. Over the ages he has brought truth and inspiration to those who are searching. His kindness, gentleness, and wisdom mark an outstanding being, radiant with love. I have no right to criticize or judge in any way this remarkable man. I need only acknowledge his fullness and greatness and divine nature. And as I think about it afterwards, this is the best I can do for any person.

As I edit this writing a month later, the impact of the whole experience returns. Different surroundings, the energy fields of different persons, have a way of eroding the grandeur of this outstanding experience. Now I am very grateful I have written up this experience, as just reading it over brings back the glory and privilege of this remarkable event.

## Chapter 12 Notes

1. Sheldrake, R. *The Presence of the Past; Morphic Resonance and the Habits of Nature*. New York: Times Books, 1988.

# Chapter 13
# Insights

In pouring over the records of our work, it took a great deal of selection to choose the accounts to include in this volume. I wished to present those which might contribute most directly to the understanding of psychedelic substances and their possible application. At the same time, I did not wish to be repetitious or too wordy.

I was left with several incidents which I felt were significant and was reluctant to leave out. I include them in this chapter for those who may enjoy more information.

*1. The marvel of self.* Related by a friend who most of her life has struggled to feel secure: Wondering why I am so unloved, I see myself as a purple flower. All the petals are people who love me. I am encouraged to look into the center of the flower. The deeper I look, the more I discover I am loved. Then follows an intriguing series of vignettes, episode after episode of life-type events. Each depicts how marvelous I am – how insightful, sensitive, perceptive, intelligent, helpful, capable, witty. I am shown every dimension of how great I am.

*2. Fear of love.* I speculate out loud on a realization I had a few days earlier: why are we so afraid of love? In the ensuing discussion, I feel the deep anguish of being separated from God. I see all the foolish things people do to try to allay this anguish – the drive for accomplishment, recognition, acquiring wealth, seducing the opposite sex. None of these bring ultimate satisfaction, which comes only from going directly to God.

*3. Mount Shasta.* Now as I look at Mount Shasta and am able to hold my mind steady, I see it as a mighty symbol of beauty and love and of enormous power. It becomes crystal clear to me that violence only begets violence. We are absolutely trapped, and strive as we may, twist and turn as we may, we can never get anywhere except through love. This is the universal law, and I have never felt so powerfully bound by it. Because this mighty mountain is an outstanding symbol of God's power, humans scramble all over it to prove that they can master it. But whatever satisfaction they get, it is only an expression of colossal arrogance until they understand that real living involves loving and brotherhood.

*4. Encountering another.* The highlight of the experience comes for me about three hours after starting, when I sit down to talk to Elnora. I become very free, open, insightful and spontaneous. I wonder why she is making such issues of what seem to be such petty things. I look at her and find myself moving deeply within her. The pain is incredible. She has had a miserable childhood, with no love or support. Her father physically abused her, and her older sister once tried to smother her to death, almost successfully. I can hold my focus and bear the pain only with the help of God's love. I hope that by holding steady, it will help her free herself. She looks back at me directly, and grows in strength and beauty. She is radiant and extremely honest. I feel and verbalize that she is a true warrior of God.

Having agreed on our understanding of karma, I ask her why she had chosen to be born into such an abusive family.[1] She's not sure, but it seems clear to me, though I prefer not to say, hoping she will discover it herself. She is extremely sensitive, easily hurt, and I feel that the inner wisdom which guides her life chose these events to permit her to learn how to develop her inner strength. I have a clear view of Christ, who would gladly pick up her burden if allowed.

I ask her if she has ever seen her own inner strength. She claims that she has, but I somehow don't feel it, at least not at the depth that would burn up all the misery she is carrying.

This encounter with Elnora felt particularly real. I felt totally free of my personality, and operating from a very profound level.

*5. Enjoying life.* After some time spent enjoying the wonderful feelings of love, I find a tendency for uncomfortable feelings to arise. I realize that there is still something deep within me that insists on turning things sour. In fact as I look at people, I often see them as miserable and uncomfortable. It occurs to me that I am projecting my own unhappiness upon them.

I decide to directly face this place within me. I hold my attention there, and encounter enormous resistance. But I maintain my attention, and the uncomfortable feeling begins to be replaced with a good one. I become more and more aware that everything is good, that everyone, despite my projections, is enjoying life far more than I realize, that enjoyment is a major aim of the unfolding processes of life. I feel better and better within myself.

*6. Feeling fully.* I am aware of walls within myself holding in feelings. I feel the wonder of allowing all of my feelings to be open to the fullest extent, regardless of what the feeling is. This is what it means to be truly alive. It is an alternate way to describe wholeness or liberation – to feel every feeling to its fullest, richest capacity. Usually we allow ourselves a mere fraction. Feeling the full depth is exquisitely satisfying, be it pleasure or pain. For being fully alive is so totally satisfying and appropriate that even pain is exquisite, for from this vantage point we see that pain is a by-product of love.

*7. Gratitude.* Fatigue is growing. I realize that I had gathered in a lot of energy, and now it is important to express it. I get up and busy myself in the kitchen. Immediately I feel worlds better. My body is extremely light and clear, and I am very energetic as I take care of tasks. I experience doing tasks and serving others as a way of expressing my gratitude for all the wonder and beauty of the day; it brings fulfillment. I again see clearly that to keep the experience alive and not fall back to previous states, it is important to fully appreciate everything that happens. This requires feeling and expressing the enormous gratitude that such realizations deserve.

*8. Reaping rewards.* We are on the shady deck watching the sky. We move into an extraordinarily beautiful part of the experience. I find that if I look at anything with complete attention, it begins to unfold and come to life. It is much more enjoyable doing this in the daylight and observing aspects of nature, rather than focusing within. I realize that my ability to do this and the clarity with which I am able to see my surroundings is a result of the work I did previously. The experience has turned to sheer beauty and enjoyment.

The next morning, after breakfast, a marvelous euphoria begins to rise within me. It mounts higher and higher until I am overcome with delight. Suddenly all the discomfort that I had gone through for years is paying off with enormous dividends. I say to Jean, "Whatever it is we have to do – face demons, pain, anger, fear, anguish, repugnance – it is all worth it to reach this marvelous level of euphoria, come unbidden and of its own accord."

I also remember past realizations that whatever time is spent directing one's gaze at God is never wasted. It is somehow stored up within, to release itself in a wonderful flow of feeling or creativity at some later, appropriate time.

*9. Partnership with God.* Moving to the sunny side of the house, we are protected by the shade of our trees and a bit of cloud cover. The view of the mountains past the green meadow is unusually striking this time of day, and for the next hour, we simply quietly relish it. I find myself preoccupied with what seems like a difference between Tim's view and my own. It is his recommendation to continue to surrender to the feelings until they resolve themselves. I feel that he considers any attempt to direct our feelings is ego. My past experiences support the view of partnership with God, where He wants a viable partner, capable of taking initiative, and providing some interest. I decide that I must test this further.

Occasionally of late I get a glimpse of a higher order, where a special kind of light seems to pervade everything, and there is an immense joy and brilliance associated with it. I feel this is contact with a higher celestial level. I start to pay attention to this, and hold my gaze steadily on it, inviting God's participation. After a while all my surroundings and my body begin to glow with love. I relax the resistances that develop as I hold my gaze, and stay focused on the love I am feeling. This love starts slowly at first, but then deepens and deepens, until I am filled with a remarkable euphoria. Everything is glowing, outside as well as within my body. I hold my mind still and simply enjoy the beauty and superb feelings.

I hold this for about an hour, and feel all charged up inside. For the first time I can ever remember, I feel that perhaps I have experienced enough euphoria.

*10. From time to eternity.* We go down to the pond and pick a nice spot under the willow tree, where we can appreciate the delicate shades of light on the water, the intimacy of growing things all around us, and a delightful sky with a great variety of cloud formations. It is peaceful to simply sit and observe. We are both still carrying some dregs of discomfort. I decide to explore what happens when I intentionally focus on love, trying hard not to direct it, but simply holding the focus so God can join me and reveal more clarity. The beauty grows, and the feelings change to euphoria. I am aware of the wonderful energy coming from Jean. I also get the sense that God is very lonely, as so few people turn their attention toward Him. But despite the lack of response and His sadness over it, He is constantly pouring out

His love to all of creation. It is a sublime feeling to pour out my love to God. As I think about love, I realize that true love gives of itself and gives generously, and asks nothing in return.

Suddenly I have an experience I have never had before. It is as if the stream of time suddenly splits, and there is a little crack in the continuity. I slip through the crack, and encounter Eternity!! In the region of Eternity is the most incredible love, far beyond any understanding of it that I have previously known. I remember the quote "Love is Eternal", and see that all true love exists on this level, which seems to be in another world beyond our ordinary world of daily affairs, and completely independent of time. It is there waiting and supporting, and ready to enter our individual world when the circumstances are right.

I remember Bartholomew telling me in a private reading that whatever we do in love always remains, is always with us to be carried on through other lifetimes. How marvelously satisfying to know that this level is there, and that we can learn to reach it and hopefully participate in it more and more. This alone gives great meaning and purpose to life. It is exquisite to sense this dimension of loving Eternity.

I again try to slip through time to re-experience it fully. It is hard to do, but I am enormously satisfied to know that it is there, that it is possible to experience it, and I know that having done it once it will be possible to enter again. What greater goal in life can one have than to learn to enter this incredible domain over and over again?

*11. Buddhism and Psychedelics.* I enter a phase which is the most important part of the experience for me. I hold the clear space within, and get an enormous appreciation of the whole Buddhist movement. These are probably the most committed people on the face of the earth in surrendering their lives totally to God, honoring God, and being channels for His light.[2] I see the enormous beauty of my meditation teacher, his dedication, and his accomplishments. Although I have been a little critical of a lot of the structure that has developed around Buddhism, I see this as relatively insignificant. It is all part of the process of developing a system to train new adepts, and have them learn enough to eventually become their own source of Being.

I look up at the mountains, seeing not only the enormous strength of the mountains, but the strength and power of the Buddhist tradition. I see how committed seekers are willing to patiently spend years and years of practice to reach the point of being touched by God, an experience that is so earthshaking and so rewarding that it is a completely sufficient reward for all of the years of patient meditation. Having just had a fresh taste, I can appreciate the full depth and power of such an experience. And this of course is what has driven the whole movement, there being adepts who have so experienced the Numinous that they inspire many others to dedicate themselves to the same search. I feel an enormous appreciation for all of the teachers and traditions that keep this movement alive and moving forward. And a great appreciation for my teacher's place in it.

So in the light of the full awareness of the importance and power of tradition and the work of all the wise ones who went before, I address the problem of understanding as clearly as possible the role of the sacraments. I can see that the use of substances represents a universal problem. There are always bright, fresh people who want to break away from tradition and establish their own approach. There is a paradox here. In one respect, a lot of such breaking away is ego-driven, the need for individuals to establish their own sense of importance. Yet it is extremely important to continue to find new and better ways.

The proper way, as I experience it, is to fully appreciate and honor those that have gone before and what they have contributed. I have often been reluctant to do this. I see that the motive for breaking away from tradition is extremely important. It is essential to be devoted to truth, and to be truly serving the Highest, which means being aware of the best outcome for everyone.

The end objective of all the practices is very clear: to establish contact with the Source. From this point on, the Source becomes the Guiding Light, and each individual becomes a sustaining, expanding channel for the Highest. It is clear that the work we have done with psychedelics has greatly accelerated this process. This has been accomplished by clearing out conditioning and repressed material, which permits more ready access to the inner core of being, the source of light. The psychedelics are practically a necessity for Western peoples, who are not going to sit for hours attempting to discipline their minds and develop sufficient power of attention to reach the higher levels of being and understanding.

With the opening provided by a good psychedelic experience, persons will more readily embrace a life of personal and spiritual growth. Disciplines aimed at such developmental goals become much more appealing. In addition, a good psychedelic experience enables a person to more readily attain rewarding states of meditation practice. The time to reach gratifying states of peace, stability, clarity, and rejuvenation is compressed, and the levels achieved are more profound.

### Chapter 13 Notes

1. Some esoteric traditions that accept reincarnation believe that between births, the individual has an opportunity to review past lives, particularly the most recent one, from a much broader, unrestricted perspective. As a result, decisions can be made about the next incarnation. Situations and events can be chosen which will best foster future growth. Since Elnora accepts this view, I could take this approach with her. See also the discussion of Past Lives Therapy, Chapter 4, pages 62-64.
2. Buddhists do not use the word God, but refer to Buddha nature, the inherent, essential ground of mind and of reality. I am sure there is no real difference. I experience this dimension in such a personal way that I deeply feel and am personally convinced of a Supreme Creator and interactive Teacher. Consequently I prefer to use the term God. My perception of God embraces all the aspects of reality taught in Buddhism. But it includes the recognition of an active Force that is not always apparent in Buddhist teachings, which often tend to be much more passive. I see this as a major difference between Western religions, which are

highly theistic, and Eastern religions. I strongly feel that each has much to offer to the other.

# Chapter 14
# Story of a Marriage

I met my first wife, Jeanette, when I was 24 years old, during World War II. Two years earlier I had been called to active duty as a reserve officer, but failed to pass the entrance medical examination or the appeal that followed. I then found employment as a civilian engineer in the Navy Department, Bureau of Ships, in Washington, D.C. for the duration of the war.

I had gone to a dance held at the local Jewish Community Center. Among the dancers I spotted an especially attractive brunette who practically took my breath away. Besides being beautiful, she was enormously poised, a trait that greatly appealed to me with my poor self-image. I found out her name, and arranged to call on her.

All went well, and soon we were dating. I knew how badly my parents wanted me to marry a Jewish girl, but I had never met one that appealed to me. Now the thought of marriage was extremely attractive, and it was only a few months until we wed.

When I look back on my first marriage, I can't believe how naive I was. I didn't know myself, I perceived very little of Jeannette's true characteristics, being content to project all kinds of fantasies upon her, and I knew nothing of male-female relationships or their potential. I was totally unprepared for marriage. There should be schools for marriage. Otherwise we are in the hands of that hard and sometimes cruel school that always teaches in the end, life itself.

I had been very anxious to marry, and proceeded compulsively. Starting with our honeymoon, I began to find out that Jeannette had many characteristics quite different than I had at first realized. But like a good Jewish husband, I made the most of it. We reared two children, a daughter, Harriet, and a son, Jerry. I settled down to a conventional life as I pursued a successful career growing up with Ampex Corporation. Ampex grew from nine people, a year after I first joined them, to 3500 employees when I left fifteen years later.

It wasn't until some twenty years later that I had my first inkling of what the possibilities might be between a man and a woman. By this time I was frequently conducting psychedelic sessions. I had the knack of soaking up all the negative feelings that were encountered by the person undergoing the experience, and I carried this around as a terrible burden. In fact, I would spend my life learning how to get free of this dross. Sitting in psychedelic sessions with clients was the hardest work I knew, and it left me continually tired.

One evening I attended a meeting in Los Angeles at the invitation of my good friend, Al Hubbard. The meeting had been arranged by his new friend Dolores, an extremely attractive, bright, sensitive, and personable young lady. She had all of the qualifications we felt were required to supervise a new branch of our Foundation in Southern California. She had gathered together a number of people who were curious about our work. The meeting was interesting, but when it was over, Dolores noticed how tired I was. She sat at one end of a sofa, and asked me to lie down and put my head in her lap. I did, but I was totally unprepared for what happened.

Almost instantly I was overcome by a sense of tranquility, and a wave of euphoria swept over me similar to the marvelous levels achieved in a good psychedelic experience. I lay there full of peace, – relaxed, content, and fulfilled. This feeling stayed with me through much of the following day.

I was astonished at what happened to me. Then I realized that what I had contacted was Feminine Essence. I had experienced the true nurturing and fulfillment that comes from a female when conditions are right.

What a remarkable discovery! At last I had a glimpse of what true male-female relations could be. No wonder there is so much fuss made about it in the world. I wondered how many men truly realize this state of affairs. I now knew that this is what we all hungered for, were desperate for. It is the lack of it that drives us into all sorts of excesses. Desperately wanting it, but pretending it is not important, we strive for mastery, for status, to be powerful, to control, to fight wars – anything but admit our crying need for the comfort of this feminine essence.

In one important sacramental experience, I realized how vital it is for our world leaders to have good marriages. For if they are happy and fulfilled as men, they can with objectivity use their best talents to address the problems of their nation. However, if they are unfulfilled, they are pushed to prove themselves in a variety of neurotic ways, with dire consequences to their country and perhaps the world.

At any rate, this was a remarkable discovery for me, and greatly influenced my life from then forward. I naturally went out immediately to prove whether this concept was correct. I sought out the company of several different women (not simultaneously) who promised to exude this cherished elixir. Sure enough, to be in their presence was wonderful and fulfilling.

I could now clearly see one of the truly important conditions to be fulfilled for a happy life. Unfortunately, this condition was not being met in my first marriage, and I never obtained enough wisdom to bring it about. Our marriage ended in divorce in 1968.

I met my current wife, Jean, in the spring of 1970. At the time, I was working as a consultant for a firm just getting established in business. This in itself was an interesting experience. The firm was run by two Christian Scientists, which greatly satisfied me as meeting the Buddhists' principle of Right Livelihood. They seemed to be wise, spiritually-oriented persons of high principle. However, this turned out to be a bitter distortion of the truth.

The president was a very clever, smooth projection of a wise, compassionate, competent business person. His very soft, low-key approach lured many investors into the company. And he was truly dedicated to God. The only trouble was that he perceived God to be himself, which totally excused all the unjust and immoral actions that he took. This led to some very interesting dilemmas within the company.

For example, the sales-training course our company was marketing to veterans was required to be an accepted part of the curriculum of an accredited college. This made it possible for the veteran to pay for the course out of Veterans Administration benefits. Our president chose a school where he had close personal contacts and which would cooperate with him. He was convinced that he could get the school approved by the Veteran's Administration.

However, he was unable to do so. Nor would he take steps to find an alternate school, so sure was he that he could get his way. This meant that we produced hundreds of product kits for a market that had no funds to pay for them. This led to the eventual demise of the company.

One day two of my co-workers, Gus and Virginia, asked me if I wished to meet an attractive young lady. Gus and Virginia had recently become husband and wife, and like so many happy couples, wished to share their joy by seeing others take advantage of their blissful state. Jean was described as an attractive, personable lady who looked very good in a bikini. This struck me as a situation worth investigating, so the three of us accepted an invitation to dinner.

As we drew up in front of the apartment house, there waiting at the head of a short flight of steps was a delightful young ten-year-old. Slim, with a very attractive body and face, delightfully feminine, was Dede, Jean's daughter. She gave a shy smile. This made me quite eager to meet her mother.

Jean turned out to be a splendid cook, quite personable, and she danced with me as a perfect partner to the music of Glenn Miller, our favorite band. I enjoyed being with her, and we began to see each other. I could feel the warmth between us, which I had come to realize is so essential, and our relationship grew into courtship, and then into marriage.

Looking back, it was a hasty marriage, as we had known each other only five months. But I was very compulsive, and once setting myself on a desired goal, I had neither the patience nor inclination to let in more data. The bottom line was that we were both lonesome and starved for companionship, and ready to commit ourselves to this relationship.

Once the need for companionship and physical needs are satisfied, other aspects of the relationship come into view. It soon became apparent that there were considerable differences in our interests, values, and aspirations.

I was an extremely serious person, putting top priority on personal growth and expansion of awareness. I was very curious, and had a powerful drive to know and understand. My accomplishment in these directions was limited only by my cowardice, which was quite appreciable. I moved in a circle of friends who shared my growth aspirations, and we spent much time examining our personal dynamics and how we could further self-understanding.

Jean had a natural talent for enjoying life, and simply accepting the flow of life. She deemed it unnecessary to analyze. Nor was she very concerned about what made things work. She was bright, but not curious to understand a number of areas. This included politics, logic, and equipment like automobiles, stereos, and VCRs. Probably at the bottom of this was a self-consciousness at not having gone further in college, and a resistance to revealing her ignorance. She covered this feeling by deciding such things were not high priority.

This of course negated many of the things I believed in, and made it difficult for her to appreciate my native gifts or accomplishments. I acutely felt this lack of acknowledgment, and in turn keenly resented her for her lack of support. On the other hand, she strongly felt my judgmentalness and criticism. She constantly felt either put down or left out of my considerations. We were continually at odds with each other, always immediately taking opposite sides of any issue. Our friends were alternately amused and annoyed at our constant bickering.

There were some ways in which we were very much alike. We were both very independent, and easily absorbed in our chosen activity. I spent as much time as I could find writing, and Jean developed considerable skill in water colors. In time she had her own studio adjacent to our house, and was producing excellent work. She had a particular flair for choosing and flowing colors, which gave an ephemeral, transcendental aura to many of her landscapes. She enjoyed very much exhibiting her work and was delighted when her works were purchased.

We both loved nature, and enjoyed hikes into the mountains. We were delighted with the location of our home, and the proximity to outstanding natural settings. When traveling, we could drive for hours with little conversation, each being absorbed in the beauty of the surrounding countryside. This joy was considerably enhanced as our perceptions were heightened through the use of psychedelics. To this day I consider it one of life's great privileges to drive in an automobile through interesting countryside, and to simply drink in the surroundings while listening to good music.

But despite these respites, our dissatisfactions continued to grow. In fact, our relationship would have been hopeless in other circumstances. We built up enormous resentments toward each other, and lost any sense of affection and mutual support. Our animosity grew to the point where it was very uncomfortable just to be with each other. Sleeping beside her at night, it often felt like a poisonous fluid was flowing from her body to mine. This seemed like a bitter toxin that pervaded my muscles and joints, causing tension, aching, and arthritis. I felt that if I didn't resolve this it would kill me.

There were times when we would tear each other down to the point that we felt it impossible to live together, and threatened to part. Yet when the reality of leaving sunk in, we decided that what we had was better than being alone, and agreed to give it another try. So cowardice was one of the things that held us together.

The other factor that kept us together, and by far the most important, was the use of the sacraments. MDMA (see Chapter 3) was a huge contributor here. In the state of grace proffered by this remarkable substance, we moved into a state of love and beauty that made the whole world a paradise. Jean called it "The Great Eraser". After a number of trials with this substance, I arrived at a list of "the usual symptoms". We would usually begin to feel the effect of the drug in about twenty minutes. Once felt, the intensity increased rapidly. There would be a rush of energy which could be a bit unsettling, except that for us the euphoric components always told us that we were heading in a good direction. At about the hour point, the rush feeling would subside, leaving us in a marvelous state approaching ecstasy. There was utter clarity of perception, with colors brilliant and everything standing out in sharp detail. Many times while starting a fire in the woodstove, I was startled by the crisp, clear, high frequency sounds made by crumpling the paper.

The outdoors was charged with energy and brilliant light, everywhere revealing the Presence of the Celestial Level. Everything seemed remarkably natural and at Peace, and in harmony with all else. As we looked at each other, we seemed fifteen years younger. Wrinkled skin would become smooth and very soft to the touch. An inner beauty shone forth. Within we felt whole, at peace, and pervaded by love. We were in love with everything that we saw. Everyone exuded kindness; problems evaporated. Everything seemed perfect the way it was.

The person who introduced us to this remarkable substance calls it Window. And rightly so, for it is like looking through a window at the world the way it should be, as the Creator intended it to be. Love, Peace, Beauty, Wonder, Harmony, Unity, Wisdom, Mystery. And such utter content. It was a joy to be with your companions. It didn't matter what you did or what you talked about or if you remained quiet, it was so joyful and peaceful to just be together.

While MDMA did not lend itself to introspection as readily as some other substances, it did permit a great deal of clarity and self-understanding if one were motivated to turn his/her attention in this direction. Problems were accurately perceived and their solutions apparent. There was a remarkable tendency when in this state to feel superbly whole and with no need to defend oneself. Differences with others could readily be discussed with remarkable freedom and insight.

The opportunity for defense-free communication and insight was not well utilized by Jean and me. When she was in the state of glory, she chose not to tarnish it by bringing up anything with a flavor of negativity. So we never discussed the problems between us. But it was indelibly impressed upon both of our minds how life could be. So even though a few days after such an experience we began to revert to our old habits, we still had in mind the model of what could be, and we were frequently moved to attempt to bring this model into reality. Without these exposures and the experience of the possible, I have no doubt that our marriage would have fallen apart early.

For quite a few years we were engaged in research with several of the new psychoactive agents. Our objective was to learn how a larger number of subjects would react to substances that we had found valuable in our own experiences. This kept us sharing journeys with others at a frequency of once every one to two weeks. These experiences were most rewarding and enjoyable, and greatly helped screen our private differences. And we continued to be exposed to more of our own inner dynamics and make progress in our personal growth.

I fell into a syndrome that continued for a number of years. Following the experiments with substances, I would be in an exalted state, loving and understanding. But over a period of days I would become exasperated with the dynamics going on between us, so that by the time of the next session, I was fairly loaded with resentment and hostility. I would work this off in the next experiment, often accompanied by much greater understanding.

As I grew to know myself better, I began to see that I was extremely self-centered and very much preoccupied with myself. I considered my work to be of prime value, and tended to devalue Jean's verbal contributions. I could practically feel the wall by which I shut her out. I began to see how painful this was to her. Furthermore, I became aware that it was my experiencing her feelings of pain and resentment which was the cause of much of the bad feelings I felt when around her. It began to dawn on me that in order to feel good, I needed to see to it that *she* felt good.

Another important discovery came from my feelings of disappointment in Jean. I yearned for more affection, more acknowledgment, more genuine interest. But as I looked at these feelings, I saw that I was producing the same feelings in her! I began to appreciate that it may be a cosmic law that my uncomfortable feelings are not those of the other person, but my very own. And the uncomfortable feelings arise from the way that I am treating the other person. These realizations helped a great deal in improving our relationship.

I worked very hard, it seemed to me, to overcome these difficulties and direct her more love and consideration and acknowledgment. However, I was very disappointed that I was receiving very little response from her. So my yo-yo existence continued for some time. Through sacramental experiences, I would reach stages of forgiveness and love, and all seemed well. Yet within a week or so the "cruddy" feelings would build up again. It seemed extremely difficult to become free. At times I wondered if I weren't squandering my life and well-being by being with the wrong partner. Yet as I addressed this, I realized that I had not achieved a sufficient level of love. I had been shown over and over that we are all One, that every living being is part of me, and that the welfare of any individual is my welfare. And since my goal was to achieve unconditional love and to relinquish my judgments of others, I surely had to do this with the person I was living with!! Again and again when in the highest states of being and I could feel my concerns for the whole world, the realization would come to me that it was senseless to think of helping the world if I couldn't get along with my own wife!

There were two kinds of experiences that helped correct this situation. One of the most impressive experiences I ever had with Jean was during a New Year's celebration when we were sharing a journey with Manual and Selma and three other very close friends. We had achieved a high level of realization. I looked at Jean and she was incredibly beautiful. I saw her face change from one form of femininity to another, each more wonderful that the last, the very essence of beauty, tenderness, nurturing, sensuousness. She laughed and smiled and showed me many delightful faces. I was overcome with love for her, and felt enormous gratitude and good fortune to have her as my wife.

This experience faded in a few days, and as I began in my own development to encounter deep shadow material, involving the release of deep, deep anger, it became very difficult to reexperience this vision. But I knew it was there, and had a goal toward which to work.

More profound and helpful was learning in journeys to tune into her Essence. When this was successful, I was overcome with the joy and delight of participating in her being. Often her nurturing and love would wipe away any discomfort I was experiencing, and a great love would grow between us. We could look together upon the world and experience the vast beauty, meaning, and joy. In this close contact, the joy and fulfillment was always greater than what I could experience alone. I knew that if I could learn to enter this state at will and maintain it, we would have a marvelous marriage.

With the availability of 2C-E (see Chapter 6), my personal growth and learning accelerated considerably. A characteristic of this substance with me was that intense, inner, negative feelings surfaced to consciousness. In fact, there was no escape. So I would simply stay with them until they were resolved. I found these experiences remarkably cleansing, and afterwards felt keenly rejuvenated, more than with any other substance.

As we cut back on our research work, Jean and I began to have more experiences with just the two of us. This required us to confront each other directly, and led to more rapid progress. Also, Jean was opening up a great deal, and was more willing to deal with her own personal dynamics.

For some time it was difficult for me, as much of the day I would so experience my repressed resentments that it was hard to become close. But we always managed to arrive at closeness by day's end. Change is extremely difficult, but it became more and more obvious that I had to alter these feelings of resentment. Fortunately, in time and with repeated experiences, and with the help of meditation practice, I was able to do so.

Here is a typical experience we shared together which contributed greatly to our understanding of each other and brought us closer:

> Jean joins me on the sofa, and I spend some time looking at her. I allow myself to be open and non-judgmental, and simply observe. I discern a great many things about her, and become aware of the push I exert for her to be different than she is. I drop this to simply see what she is of herself. At one point I realize that we are each every man and every woman, and become fascinated with how we choose certain faces and dynamics to present to each other. In a sense it doesn't make any difference who your partner is, if you can learn to present to each other the most interesting and desirable aspects.
>
> I become aware that there are flaming sexual energies within us both. I can see that Jean has generated enormous resentment toward me for frustrating her energies by being so absorbed within myself and not fully expressing myself sexually. I in turn do not choose to express myself completely because of my resentments over certain aspects of our relationship. So I take refuge in seeking satisfaction from inner feelings generated by more deeply contacting my inner being. We can do a great deal for each other by freeing these energies and expressing them to each other.

As I look over the various facets we can present each other, I wonder if I can see the highest aspects of Jean. I carefully watch, not pushing, and her beauty begins to reveal itself. For a while I am filled with the grace of the essence of her being, manifested in a wonderful radiance. This is most satisfying, but not easy to keep present.

An underlying feeling of extreme tiredness has pervaded both Jean and me throughout the day. When we decide that our groveling time is over, we put on some music and dance. It is remarkable how the flow of energy carries us to new dimensions, releasing wonderful feelings and understandings that do not come while lying down and breathing through the discomforts. This is a compelling experience.

At last we reached the stage where we began to genuinely enjoy each other. Forgiveness became real, and we committed ourselves to treating each other with kindness and concern. The result was a growth in the energy flow between us which became sustaining and energizing.

. . . . . . .

One of the very intriguing developments is how, despite our differences, the sensual pleasures of lovemaking grew with time. Starting a few years ago, I experienced a reduction in potency. I ascribed this to advancing age, the possible effects of a prostate operation, or even the claim made by some of the adverse effects of a vasectomy as one grows old. All of these concerns evaporated as Jean and I accepted each other and moved into real caring and intimacy.

I remain convinced that the most significant factor involving sensual pleasure is the emotional closeness of the partners. Hostility and resentment are real killers of profound sexual enjoyment.

One incident stands out as an illustration of the dynamics involved in achieving closeness. Jean and I spent a week in a meditation retreat with Alan Wallace, our teacher of Tibetan Buddhist meditation. My meditative experiences improved considerably, as well as my ability to be at peace in the moment.

Jean left shortly after the retreat for a week in the Bay Area visiting her daughter and grandchildren. During her absence I experienced the greatest contentment ever while alone. Nevertheless, I was eagerly looking forward to Jean's return.

I was delighted to see her when she arrived home. I immediately felt the warmth of her presence. But then I was suddenly struck with a sickening sensation. The heavy, miserable feelings I used to feel in her presence that had plagued me for years were back in full force! This was a disastrous blow. I felt I had made enormous progress in dissipating these feelings. Now I must rethink my progress, my goals, and decide about the future. I certainly didn't want to continue life carrying this burden. But I also didn't want to live alone. Was there any way to solve this problem?

On my daily afternoon walk with our two dogs, I prayed deeply about it. I saw that there was a lot I was still demanding of Jean, hoping that she would cooperate to achieve the remarkable state of union between us I knew was possible. It was clear that my intensity and manipulating were creating the discomfort. The union I so fervently wished for necessitated the agreement of both parties. I couldn't force her to do it. I had to let her proceed in her own way at her own pace. This realization eased my state of being considerably.

I slept alone that night and the next morning Jean joined me in bed. Immediately I felt the miserable feelings as though they were flowing directly from her body into mine like toxins. I simply relaxed, accepted it, and stayed with it. It continued to grow in intensity until it was unbearable. I prayed desperately to be shown a way out, or to at least understand what the feeling was.

I began to feel a focus of a sharp pain, and immediately willed myself into it. Simultaneously I remembered that when I woke up in the middle of the night I was on the edge of an extremely frightening experience. This also had been plaguing me for years, and especially as I had grown older. I often woke up in the middle of the night in deep, agonizing, inexplicable feelings, the worst of the whole day. I had grown used to them, and had dropped my concern about them, since once I was up and around they disappeared, and I was able to conduct myself in a comfortable and often joyous state.

But this morning as I experienced the sharp pain and remembered my nocturnal miseries, the two came together. I suddenly realized I was experiencing deeply within Jean the enormous pain of being unloved. The feeling was a desperate, anguished cry for love that soon spread throughout all of humanity. Humans everywhere, including myself, are agonized at the emptiness of our inner being.

I saw the need to fill this emptiness in Jean with love. I began to flow love to her, and as I did, God joined me and supplied His infinite reservoir of love. I could feel love flowing into all the compartments of her being. The miserable feelings dissolved and I was feeling only the wonder of God's love, and His capacity to wipe away the deepest suffering.

I realized this would be still more effective by expressing love through physical lovemaking. We came together in the most sensuous, wonderful, love-filled experience that I can remember. My mind was filled with Jean completely, and I did everything possible to convey tenderness, pleasure, and nurturing. It was an outstanding experience.

Then I realized I wished to be nurtured too, and I felt her nurturing essence begin to fill me. The joy and pleasure reached tremendous new heights as we were both being filled. Then suddenly the nurturing stopped flowing into me, and despite the most pleasurable stimulation, I lost my potency. I was yearning for completion, but the energy wasn't available.

I relaxed and I thought, "This is really karma". For many times in the past I had been completed and fulfilled when Jean was not. Now it was my turn to be left unfulfilled. But the yearning rapidly subsided as we relaxed into the joy of being together and sharing our warmth and love. And there would soon be a next time.

A very interesting thing that Jean shared with me was that at the beginning when I was sinking into misery, she was having the most enjoyable time ever being next to me. It was because I was so relaxed, and not trying or pushing!

The use of the sacraments played an important role in the progress of our lovemaking. The sacraments were very effective in amplifying sensuousness and intimacy, so that lovemaking continued to grow in pleasure and satisfaction. While the amplification of pleasure is highest while under the influence, much of the enhancement becomes permanent.

In the early stages of our marriage, when we each held considerable anger toward the other, the joy of lovemaking would often be followed by languidness or tiredness. Sometimes this would even get as strong as revulsion. Sexual hunger is a powerful drive, and sexual satisfaction is one of life's greatest pleasures. So lovemaking continues in many relationships long past the time of true affection. There are no doubt countless marriages in which the sex drive is the only thing that holds the couple together, and may be the only bit of pleasure derived from the relationship.

In my own case, during the time when I yearned for more understanding and affection, I felt I was violating my integrity by making love to a partner for whom I felt no affection. This created enormous self-hatred.

Our marriage improved substantially as I began to appreciate Jean's true nature. I caught up with my personal dynamic of putting Jean down instead of facing the very difficult task of changing my deeply ingrained habits. These habits centered on my self-absorption, shutting Jean out and not acknowledging her, and my unwillingness to relinquish my judgmental, critical attitude, as well as my resentments.

Much of my resentment was grounded in a deep, powerful self-hatred which I did not care to confront. It is much easier to project self-hatred onto those around you. I think it is a psychological truth that those to whom we are the closest and can therefore trust the most are often the target of our most severe projections.

My inability to hold on to the superior states of well-being that resulted from the use of the sacraments and from good meditations forced me to realize I had to break these habits. As I was able to do so, true affection began to grow.

As we opened to each other, it became possible to experience closer and closer the core of the other's being. This made it possible to feel a deeper, more profound love. It kept increasing in intensity until it became nurturing and fulfilling.

I began experiencing more frequently the Feminine Essence mentioned earlier in this chapter. I believe that men can perceive this as a nurturing, enrapturing nectar that fills us with consummate fulfillment, a peace and ecstasy that is beyond describing. It is what our nature calls for, yearns for. And it is available only by opening ourselves completely to our partner, allowing love to penetrate our being without reservation.

Such opening to one another allows the essence of our beings to bond deeply, to unite us in the most heart-felt love. And this in turn remarkably enhances lovemaking. This intimacy not only heightens the joy of all physical contact, but results in a healing, nurturing exchange of energy that charges us for the day. In the glow of such fulfillment, it is easy to see the remarkable beauty of life in all that surrounds us.

While many of the world's spiritual disciplines lay a path to ultimate fulfillment through solitude, I must report that every step that I have been able to accomplish has been a great deal more fulfilling in harmony with a loving partner. In view of the crippling obstacles that once polluted Jean's and my relationship, it is most satisfying to discover the affection and support that open the door to higher appreciation of the wonders around us. Again and again I express my gratitude for the intuition that helped me recognize that the difficulties were within myself, and for the forces that helped me gather the determination to keep working on the factors that kept us apart. Now there is the gratifying satisfaction of having a partner who is a true companion, a true helpmate – one who makes it possible to appreciate the blessings of life. This is living at its utmost.

# Chapter 15
# Culmination

Writing this book has been a very rewarding enterprise. Reviewing the raw material from which this book was drawn has driven home how abundantly I have been blessed – for the outstanding experiences I have had, the wonderful people that I have met and shared with, the thrill of entering new dimensions of understanding, and the joy of realizing how wonderful life can be as important truths are accepted and acted upon.

Before recounting what I consider to be valuable realizations from my work with psychedelics, I wish to address a few issues that may be of concern.

The first is the issue of addiction. I was rather shocked one morning when a good psychologist friend told me over the phone, "Myron, you are addicted to psychedelics!"

I hung up the phone, looked out the window at one of my favorite mountain peaks, and pondered this question. The answer came flooding in. "Thank God!" I could profoundly see how blessed I have been, what remarkable experiences I have had, how I have been privileged to learn priceless information concerning many aspects of reality, how I have learned of the unspeakable wonder of Divine Love, and am even learning to manifest it a bit. I gave thanks to be so blessed, and grateful that I had had the good sense to make important, if difficult, choices: the choice to seek and learn, the choice to surrender to whatever reality wished to manifest, and that most challenging choice of all – to put what I had learned into living action. With these choices there is no end to exploring, to learning, to loving, to enjoying. So yes, I am addicted, just as I am addicted to sex, good food, good music, and the company of good friends. I will always go back for more whenever appropriate.

Can others become addicted? No doubt. There are addictive personalities who can become addicted to almost anything. These most likely are the ones who are starved for contact with their innermost being. The separation from one's soul is, I believe, the most painful thing humankind can experience. Because of the agony, we are extremely adept at shielding this pain from conscious awareness. But this hidden pain demands mitigation. So we will look for any outlet to try to assuage this feeling of inner emptiness, as I have mentioned in several reports in this volume. Most devices we seek are attempts to assure ourselves of our inherent worth, a search that can only be genuinely fulfilled by discovery of our true inner nature.

Many, no doubt, have found temporary solace in psychedelic substances. But only true, rich encounters with our inner being can dissolve the pain and permit a fresh, immediate understanding of life and show the appropriate way to a joyful, fulfilling life.

Rewarding outcomes require good preparation. Important factors assuring good results include honest intent, good information, sound teachers and guides, and a good peer group who will candidly reflect feelings and perceptions. A powerful influence for continuing development is the Buddhist custom of committing oneself to the welfare and happiness of all beings.

Is there any physical deterioration from the use of psychedelic substances? With intelligent use I have found that they convincingly produce the opposite.

My own mental state has cleared up steadily as I have worked through and abandoned the inner dross I had accumulated most of my life from painful betrayals, repressed painful memories, deep conditioning, and living out of harmony with my true self. While at age seventy-three I am beginning to notice some memory loss, especially as regards to names, in most other ways my mind has gained clarity and I can think more productively than ever before. I now often experience the flow of ideation and the broadening of concepts that used to be available only under the influence of a sacrament. I have to admit to being amused when, after I have shared with others my tendency toward forgetfulness, they say, "Yeah, that's happening more and more to me too!" And they are usually fifteen to twenty years younger than I.

I am still in excellent physical health, and very much enjoy a good hike at least once a week, gaining a thousand feet or more in elevation. While many of my friends recommend vitamins, antioxidants, smart pills, etc., I find the sacraments the best overall vitamins for producing rejuvenation, vitality, and zest for life.

I have already discussed sexual satisfaction in Chapter 15, Story of a Marriage.

With all of these attributes, wouldn't you think that pleasure-happy American people would rush to embrace these substances? No. The reasons are quite clear, and powerful. To achieve these results requires honesty and fortitude. It requires the willingness to abandon pet ideas and the yearning for superiority, so that new, vital information can be learned. It requires a willingness to face up to the errors of the past. And if one is not willing to abandon harmful or destructive behavior, psychedelic experiences can leave one more uncomfortable than before imbibing.

So these substances work best for honest persons who truly wish to grow, who fully appreciate life and are looking for additional ways to participate in it and express their gratitude. Such people have no doubt already discovered useful frameworks for their development.

The above requirements for productive outcomes may rule out large numbers of people. All we ask of them is that they not be disturbed if they don't understand. We simply ask to please let those who wish to dig more deeply into wisdom and serve life more fully to be allowed to do so. In the end, all will benefit!

As I review my own use of the sacraments, I am aware that much of my life has been a struggle to become free of ponderous weights that seem to drag like heavy anchors. But as the anchors were recognized and cut free, and more importantly, as I recognized and accepted the forces in the universe that are there to pick up the weights and cut the entangling ropes, I was able to achieve greater freedom and joy.

Now as I survey the planet, I can see wonderful places of light and beauty, but also many shadows, some of which are very grim. But I have learned it is possible to live more and more in the sunlight. I have glimpsed intimations of the brilliant, heavenly light that suffuses all – a light so radiant, so healing, so completely full of love that it is sheer ecstasy to be immersed in it. In my highest moments, I can momentarily become this light. From this plane of existence the celestial light shines wherever I look, in every living creature, in every created object.

I can see that when immersed in the celestial light, life is completely transformed. As Brother Lawrence describes in *The Practice of the Presence of God*,[1] the most menial task can be irradiated with this heavenly light that it is our privilege to emit. The most irksome task can be an act of worship and celebration.

I am aware of the possibility of participating ever more deeply in the transcendental light. I know that it becomes more constant as I commit myself to it and learn how to allow it to manifest. A vital part of this learning is seeing the light manifested in others. It is eminently satisfying to focus on the happiness and welfare of others.

There are some serious spiritual seekers who see this earthly plane of existence as a form of purgatory, where we learn what we must and then leave it behind. There is supposedly a much superior plane of existence beyond this material world.

While this may be so and some find this notion compelling, I am presently more enthralled with the potential of existence on this earthly plane. Like Sri Aurobindo, I see the goal as bringing the Divine into the world. I am convinced that this worldly level of existence was created for an important reason. Humankind is in the very primitive stages of awakening; we have a great deal further to go in order to discover and realize the full, exciting potential of earthly existence. I see enormous opportunities for us to develop ourselves, to incorporate in our beings and actions more and more Divine love, to transform ourselves and the world into a paradise – the true Kingdom of God.

It doesn't mean that we have to abandon any of the activities we are now engaged in, except for those that interfere with the well-being and happiness of ourselves and others. We can learn to do most all the things we now do, except with real joy, interest, and excitement. We can discover and create new things even more exciting and fulfilling.

It may be that mankind has become too depraved to allow the Kingdom to manifest on a broad scale. But it is hard for me to see how anyone with true understanding can avoid dedicating him/herself to the goal of liberation for everyone. After all, we are all One, and I cannot reach true liberation until all have been liberated. Yes, I can free myself, but there will always be that area of pain that shall exist as long as another human being somewhere is hurting. I may learn to turn my attention away from it, but it will always be there when I look. I am confident that as each individual becomes free, I will experience more freedom.

I agree that we must surrender, that we must learn to die. The Buddhists are right – our desires and investments are the prime causes of suffering. As we relinquish our investments, our pet ideas, our repressed feelings, our ignorance, and as we acknowledge our shadow, it becomes possible to experience larger dimensions of ourself. These other dimensions are enormously gratifying, ultimately rooted in indescribable love.

My personal experiences have helped me appreciate the vastness of the love God holds for each of us, and the incredible love we can learn to pass on to others. Some say that for true liberation the self must be annihilated. But so far, even though I have witnessed the dimensions of my being expand to infinite proportions, including the entire created universe, I have always found that I am still here, faced with the incredible mystery of the vastness of myself and the wonder of Divine Glory that cares for me and fills me.

I have much to learn and realize and hopefully contribute in this exciting enterprise. When I need to learn more, to gain greater understanding, I know that the best thing to do is to relinquish myself to my Teacher, open myself to new experience, and allow myself to be shown what wishes to manifest. I am confident that when it is important for me to take another step, it shall happen in this manner. I hope to have the courage to stay open and to follow where I am led. In the meantime, I am enormously grateful for what has transpired to date.

In mulling over all of this and watching the ups and downs in my state of being as I have progressed through these various experiences, I have been repeatedly surprised about how much of the responsibility I have had to shoulder. I had always thought that if I were surrendered and open, I would be filled with love and function perfectly. Instead I often lapsed into an uncomfortable state of passive detachment. Time and again I have been reminded that I have already been shown the answer to the problem facing me, and it is up to me to act on it. I have repeatedly found it necessary to deepen my resolve, to deepen my intention, to wake up, to pay attention. Intentionality is a most important requirement of the committed life.

But equally important is learning how to be open and to surrender, to be perfectly still, to listen from deeply within the soul. I find that it is in the appropriate balance of these dynamics – surrendering to discover new wisdom, and taking responsibility for action – that life moves forward most satisfactorily.

When I am whole, there is no distinction between God and myself. Such concepts disappear, and life flows with an indescribable, spontaneous grace. But in my present state many things pull me down, and I cannot maintain such a state of wholeness. When I relapse, the most effective means I have found to reestablish my true self is my understanding of being a partner with God, and of how this partnership works. This is a partnership, as I understand it, that every being must work out for him/herself. Full partnership requires a comprehensive understanding of the remarkable role that we have been created to fill, and how unstintingly our loving endeavors are supported. Short of full union with God, it is in this partnership that life reaches its most glorious, sublime, exciting, purely joyous heights.

It is my earnest hope that these pages have revealed enough information to inspire others to start or deepen their commitment to the path of true fulfillment.

### Chapter 15 Notes

1. Brother Lawrence. *Practice of the Presence of God.* New York: Walker and Co. 1985.

# Appendix I
# Foundation Papers

The following are published papers resulting from research conducted at the International Foundation for Advanced Study:

Sherwood, J. N., Stolaroff, M., and Harman, W. W. "The Psychedelic Experience – A New Concept in Psychotherapy". *Journal of Neuropsychiatry* 4: 69-80, 1962.

Savage, C., Stolaroff, M., Harman, W. W., and Fadiman, J. "Caveat! The Psychedelic Experience". *Journal of Neuropsychiatry* 5: 4-5, 1963.

Mogar, R., and Savage, C. "Personality Change Associated with Psychedelic (LSD) Therapy: A Preliminary Report". *Psychotherapy* 1: 154-162, 1964.

Savage, C., Savage, E., Fadiman, J., and Harman, W. W. "LSD: Therapeutic Effects of the Psychedelic Experience". *Psychological Reports* 14: 111-120, 1964.

Savage, C., and Stolaroff, M.J. "Clarifying the Confusion Regarding LSD-25". *The Journal of Nervous and Mental Disease* 140: 218-221, 1965.

Savage, C., Fadiman, J., Mogar, R., and Allen, M.H. "The Effects of Psychedelic (LSD) Therapy on Values, Personality, and Behavior". *International Journal of Neuropsychiatry* 2: 241-254, 1965.

Harman, W. W., McKim, R. H., Mogar, R. E., Fadiman, J., and Stolaroff, M. "Psychedelic Agents in Creative Problem-Solving: A Pilot Study". *Psychological Reports* 19: 211-227, 1966.

# Appendix II
## Degree of Intensity Scale

Excerpted from "A Protocol for the Evaluation of New Psychoactive Drugs in Man" by Alexander T. Shulgin, L. Ann Shulgin, and Peyton Jacob, III, published in *Methods and Findings in Experimental and Clinical Pharmacology* 8(5): 313-320, 1986.

- There is no effect noted, of any nature, that can be ascribed to the drug in question.

+/- There is a move away from baseline, but there is not necessarily a conviction that it is drug-related.

+1 There is a real effect, and the duration but not the nature of the content can be discerned. The "alert" has progressed into something unmistakable.

+2 There is an unmistakable effect, and both the duration and the nature of the effect can be stated. At +2, one might be able to answer a telephone sensibly, but would most probably choose not to attempt to do so. One could drive a car with much care, but would wisely choose to do so only in a life-and-death emergency. Cognitive factors are largely intact, and much of the drug's effect could be suppressed if the need should arise.

+3 This is the level of maximum intensity of drug effect. The full potential of the drug has been realized. Its character can be spelled out and the chronological patterns to be expected are defined.

+4 A special designation for "peak experience" in the terminology of Abe Maslow. This is a serene and magical state which is largely independent of what drug is used, if a drug at all, and moreover, cannot be repeated at will with a repetition of the experiment. It is the extraordinary place, that one-of-a-kind, mystical or religious experience that will never be forgotten. This is not to imply in any way that it is more than, or comparable to, the +3. It is simply in a class by itself, and has no suggestion of quantitative value.

# Appendix III
# Procedure

Experiments were conducted in a relaxed, informal setting as described by Shulgin, Shulgin, and Jacobs.[1] They were often conducted over a weekend. This gave the opportunity for those participating to get together the evening before, get acquainted if necessary, and learn about the substance to be tried and its characteristics. It also gave the opportunity to share concerns and aspirations, as well as determine individual dose levels from the data available.

Participants chosen for research with new compounds (with the exception of MDMA) had previous experience with psychedelics, were stable personalities with whom it was easy to establish good rapport, and were unlikely to be frightened or overwhelmed by the surfacing of unconscious material. They were assessed to have a favorable "set", a requirement for a fruitful psychedelic experience. The following description of the effect of set and setting on the experience is excerpted from my paper in the journal *Gnosis:*[2]

> Set and setting have been widely recognized as the two most important factors in undertaking a psychedelic experience. Of these set has the greatest influence.
>
> As the drug opens the door to the unconscious, huge spectrums of possibilities present themselves. Just how one steers through this vast maze depends mostly upon set. Set includes the contents of the personal unconscious, which essentially is the record of all one's life experiences. It includes the walls of conditioning which determine the freedom with which one can move through various vistas. Another important aspect of set consists of one's values, attitudes, and aspirations. These will influence the direction of attention and determine how one deals with the material encountered.
>
> In fact one can learn a great deal by accepting and reconciling oneself with uncomfortable material. Resisting this discomfort, on the other hand, can greatly intensify the level of pain, leading to disturbing, unsatisfactory experiences, or even psychotic attempts to escape. This latter dynamic is largely responsible for the medical profession's view of these materials as psychotomimetic. Surrender, acceptance, gratitude, and appreciation can result in continual opening, expansion, and fulfillment.
>
> Setting, or the environment in which the experience takes place, can also greatly influence the experience, since subjects are often very suggestible under psychedelics. Inspiring ritual, a beautiful natural setting, stimulating art work, and interesting objects to examine can focus one's attention on rewarding areas. Most important of all is an experienced, compassionate guide who is very familiar with the process. His mere presence establishes a stable energy field that helps the subject remain centered. The guide can be very helpful should the subject get stuck in uncomfortable places, and can ask intelligent questions that will help resolve difficulties, as well as suggesting fruitful directions of exploration that the subject might have otherwise overlooked. The user will also find that simply sharing what is happening with an understanding listener will produce greater clarity and comfort. Finally, a good companion knows that the best guide is one's own inner being, which should not be interfered with unless help is genuinely needed and sought.

On the day of the session, the drug was taken on an empty stomach. Participants were free to follow their own inclinations. They could gather in groups and chat, or wander into private rooms or around the grounds for private exploration.

The surrounding countryside provided beautiful vistas, looking over granite rock formations, a green meadow, and towering mountains. There were many interesting spots to sit and drink in nature. "The flat rock" was a favorite of mine I often referred to in reports of experiences. It was a very large, flat-surfaced rock that sat above the surrounding landscape, and was surrounded by growing bushes and shrubs. It looked over a green meadow filled with grazing cattle, and offered views of interesting granite rock piles and abruptly rising high mountains. The view was commanding and revealed much of the beauty, mystery, and wonder of the high desert.

Another favorite I called my "meditation rock". It was a well-formed seat permitting reclining, atop an isolated, tall rock pile. It had the advantage of a 360°, unrestricted view of the surrounding countryside. It was an ideal spot for contemplating natural environments.

Except in special cases where individuals had specifically asked for help or guidance, each person was left to explore the experience in his or her own way. Soft drinks and snacks were available. Groups usually found it worthwhile to join together for mutual discussion after they had sufficient time for private investigation. A good music system was also available, and many greatly enjoyed the increased enhancement often experienced with music. Music can be very inspiring in encouraging releasing to the experience and opening the door for new levels of exploration.

The day following the experiences provided time for the participants to share and discuss their individual journeys.

### Appendix III Notes


1. Shulgin, A. T.; Shulgin, A.; & Jacob, P. III. "A Protocol for the Evaluation of New Psychoactive Drugs in Man". *Methods and Findings in Experimental and Clinical Pharmacology* 8(5): 313-320, 1968.
2. Stolaroff, M. J., 1993. "Using Psychedelics Wisely". *Gnosis, a Journal of the Western Inner Traditions* No. 26, Winter 1993, pp. 26-30.

## Appendix IV
## The Nature of the Self

My large number of experiences ingesting psychedelic substances has shed a great deal of light on the nature of the psyche and the nature of the human mind. The raw data can be interpreted in a variety of ways, depending upon the viewpoint of the observer. Information learned under the influence of a psychedelic is somewhat suspect, as it has been demonstrated time and again that perceptions are highly colored by the values, beliefs, and experience of the observer. Such pre-dispositions can even be reinforced by the action of the drug. An additional consideration is that the intensity of focus and clarity permitted by the action of the chemical highly emphasizes the significance of the point of focus in relation to other data.

However, with honest searching and the willingness to investigate a variety of viewpoints, a procedure can be developed for validating experiences. It will no doubt incorporate many aspects of the advice for contemplatives in the Catholic Church.[1] Revelations are to be regarded with suspicion until verified by practical, proven methods. This includes tests of logic, appropriateness, and the assumption that if a revelation is true, it will repeat itself. The contributions of an informed peer group are invaluable.

Based on a large number of my own experiences and those of others, I have arrived at the following view regarding the nature of the human psyche. The largest area to be explained, and what is least familiar to Westerners, is the nature of the human unconscious mind.

I am convinced through my own observations that the most important action of a psychedelic chemical is to dissolve the barrier between the conscious and unconscious mind. This potentially provides access to all our forgotten memories, repressed feelings, hidden motives, drives, values, and habits as recognized by Sigmund Freud.

In addition, a great deal of other information has been revealed which supports the view that the famous Swiss psychiatrist Carl G. Jung shas been the most accurate assessor of the human psyche. Many have discovered the worlds of symbols that Jung postulated as well as the various human archetypes that he described.

Probably the most important concept of Jung's that has been verified is that of the Collective Unconscious. This concept states that if each of us as individuals goes deeply enough into our own unconscious, we reach a vast, infinite sea that is common to all of us, and consequently joins us all. This explains why such extra-sensory phenomena as telepathy and clairvoyance are possible. It also is the basis of the harmony and oneness that is so often described in psychedelic experiences.

The Collective Unconscious is infinite and includes every possible aspect of mind. This accounts for the enormous variety of symbols, imagery, memories ancient and recent, and visits to other lands, times, and events that are so frequently reported in psychedelic journeys. The concept of the Collective

Unconscious is a counterpart of Universal Mind, which is a tenet of many esoteric traditions. As such, it contains all wisdom and all experience.

Some esoteric traditions hold that there is such a thing as the Akashic Records (see Chapter 4, Note 2). Here every action, feeling, and thought of every living creature is recorded, and is available to each individual through his own unconscious. That would logically make it part of the Collective Unconscious.

Within the Collective Unconscious is the Source of all being, which includes the origin of natural laws and all material objects and living forms. This Source is also the genesis of the prolific imagery encountered in dreams, trance states, and psychedelic journeys, and is the root of wisdom, intuition, and creativity. My experience of the Source is that it is at the core or essence of everything created. This core is the life force, the radiant energy that suffuses and sustains all living creatures and all of creation. I have sometimes perceived this as the Central Furnace.

To approach this core is to approach the center of energy, an unbelievably brilliant light that is Love Manifest. It is so bright and unimaginably beautiful that it is almost impossible to gaze upon. Mystics have claimed that it is a light brighter than a thousand suns. Meister Eckhart has stated that all the privations humanly bearable would amount to naught for the privilege of looking into this Face.[2] We can learn that the Source of this love cares for each and every one of us, and everything in creation beyond anything we can imagine. And we as humans have the possibility of uniting with this core, becoming the source of this unbridled light and love and unending wisdom.

This state has been given various names. In Western religions – Judaism and Christianity – it is called Union with God. The Buddhists, who have probably explored the nature of mind more extensively than any people on earth, call it realizing one's Buddha Nature. In such a state we are immersed in the ground of being, the ground of reality, the ground of the mind. Alternate Eastern terms for such a state are enlightenment or liberation. When we become truly enlightened or liberated, then we merge with our true inner nature or Buddha nature. Liberation comprises freedom from concepts and conditioning, so that we may freely attend any aspect of Universal Mind or Buddha nature. Excellent descriptions aimed at shedding light on the subjective experience of such a realization are given by Sogyal Rimpoche in his powerful book *The Tibetan Book of Living and Dying*.[3]

We are told by the great teachers, particularly Buddha himself, the Enlightened One, that enlightenment is a state that is potentially within us all, and can be achieved in this lifetime. It is the birthright of every human being. The twentieth century Indian mystic Ramana Maharshi claims that the only reason we are not enlightened is that we do not know that we are already enlightened.

If such a magnificent state exists, and if the inner light is so profoundly intense, then why don't we experience it? We are obviously shielded from this light by powerful, impacted layers of screens that we do not understand. This is the residue in our unconscious mind.

In examining myself, I find that my inner core is surrounded by layer upon layer of conditioning. This conditioning is formed by repressed feelings, false ideas and beliefs, needs, stresses, drives, desires, and habits. Much of this material blocks the expression of the true life force, which is love. The more traumatic and painful were early life experiences, the more impacted and heavily defended are these layers of conditioning. The solidity of the deepest layers of conditioning, and the difficulty of working through them, are discussed in the latter part of Chapter 2, pages 37 and 38.

A very important part of these occluding layers is that powerful, hidden part of ourselves that Jung calls our Shadow – all of the information that we have a vested interest in hiding from ourselves. Unfortunately, our Shadow controls a great deal of our energy and causes us to behave in ways of which we are not aware. The greatest problem is that we project our Shadows onto others, and thereby make other persons the cause of our difficulties. Reconciling the contents of our Shadow, and taking full responsibility for ourselves, would accomplish an enormous amount in removing human differences and achieving world harmony.

There are a variety of practices that have been developed throughout the world to discard this blocking conditioning and release our true, inner self. In America, the most recognized way of seeking help to become free of the accumulations which make life unpleasant or unsatisfactory is to consult a professional therapist. A good therapist can help us understand inappropriate unconscious patterns and help us get free of them. It is often a very long and sometimes agonizing process.

In the East a great variety of meditation practices have been developed to accomplish the goal of enlightenment or liberation. These practices are quite time-consuming, and this can be a long, arduous path. But once the benefits begin to be tasted, it is difficult to turn away from this course.

The same things can be accomplished by the informed use of psychedelics, with some powerful additional advantages. An outstanding characteristic of psychedelics when properly used is that they dissolve the boundary between the conscious and unconscious mind, thereby giving us direct access to unconscious material. This can reveal much that is helpful for rapid personal growth.

Another prime advantage is that under favorable circumstances, psychedelics can let us discover our inner core, thereby opening us to grace. Grace can come in the form of wisdom, insight, and understanding. Its powerful light of love is healing and rejuvenating. The knowledge and certainty it can bring gives confidence, direction, and purpose to our lives. Grace brings energy and inspiration. Once the door is opened to grace, it can be a continuing source of guidance and nourishment.

### Appendix IV Notes

1. Poulain, A. *Graces of Interior Prayer, A Treatise on Mystical Theology*. London: Routledge and Kegan Paul Limited, 1951. In this most comprehensive and well-

documented treatment of mystical prayer, Poulain devotes four chapters to revelations, covering descriptions, dangers of illusions, how to judge revelations, and rules of conduct, pp. 299-396.

2. Oliver Davies, ed. *The Rhineland Mystics*. New York: Crossroads, 1990, p. 34: "If someone were to possess a whole kingdom, or all the goods of the earth, and were to give it all up for the sake of God and were to become one of the poorest people who live anywhere on earth, and if God were then to give them as much suffering as he has ever given anyone, for all his days; if then God were to allow him to glimpse his nature as it exists in this power, his joy would be so great that he would feel that all this suffering and all this poverty had been too little."
3. Sogyal Rinpoche. *The Tibetan Book of Living and Dying*. San Francisco: Harpers, 1992. See the section entitled The View (seeing from the liberated state), pp. 152-159.